To Noelle and Norma

K. York Chynn
Nathaniel Finby

Manual of Cranial Computerized Tomography

146 figures, 1 table,
6 color plates, 1982

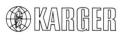 **KARGER**

S. Karger
Basel · München · Paris · London · New York · Sydney

The Authors

K. York Chynn, MD, FACR,
is Clinical Professor of Radiology, College of Physicians
and Surgeons, Columbia University, as well as Attending
Radiologist and Head of Neuroradiology, St. Luke's Hospital Center, New York, New York.

Nathaniel Finby, MD, FACR,
is Professor of Clinical Radiology, College of Physicians
and Surgeons, Columbia University; Attending Radiologist
and Chairman, Department of Radiology, St. Luke's-
Roosevelt Hospital Center; and Consultant to St. Barnabas
Hospital for Chronic Disease, New York, New York.

National Library of Medicine, Cataloging in Publication
    Chynn, K. York
    Manual of cranial computerized tomography / K. York Chynn,
    Nathaniel Finby.—Basel; New York: Karger, 1982
    1. Skull—radiography 2. Tomography, X-Ray Computer I. Finby,
    Nathaniel II. Title
    WE 705 C564m
    ISBN 3–8055–3432–9

© Copyright 1982 by S. Karger AG, P.O. Box,
    CH–4009 Basel (Switzerland)
    Printed in the United States of America

Contents

Acknowledgments

Dr. Nathaniel Finby wishes to express his sincere appreciation to:

> Robert A. Phillips, PhD
> Bureau of Radiologic Health
> HFX-460 U.S. Department of Health and
>   Consumer Service
> Food and Drug Administration
> Rockville, Maryland

who co-authored chapter I of this manual.

Dr. Kuo-York Chynn wishes to specifically acknowledge Michael E. Mawad, MD of Columbia Presbyterian Medical Center, New York for his skillful assistance with the preparation of the color illustrations used in this manual. Furthermore, Drs. Ina Altman and William I. Shaw have shared some of the clinical neuroradiologic responsibilities, and have made the undertaking of this project possible.

The authors express their gratitude to the entire attending staff of St. Luke's Roosevelt Hospital Center. The staff, whose members are too numerous to be listed here, referred their patients for the studies that are illustrated in this book. Most neurologic examinations were carried out by our attending neurologists, Drs. Carl W. Braun, Sidney E. Bender, Gary Korenman, Donald G. Rawlinson, Daniel A. Alkaitis, Linda R. Lewis, Thomas C. Guthrie and Lewis Travis. All neurologic operations were performed by our attending neurosurgeons, Drs. Robert W. Schick, James E. O. Hughes and George V. DiGiancinto Jr.

The authors of this book thank E.R. Squibb & Sons, Inc. for underwriting the cost of reproducing the color illustrations used in this manual.

Preface

Computed tomography has been in existence for more than a decade. The first installation was in October of 1971, at Atkinson Morley Hospital, Wimbledon, London. During this period, the wide applications of cranial computed tomography were established, and are now well known to qualified neuroradiologists.

However, requests for computed tomography are usually initiated by house physicians or attending physicians from various subspecialities, who are not completely familiar with the capability and the limitations of this new diagnostic modality. Furthermore, radiologists in training and general radiologists are frequently consulted regarding perplexing CT images. Since the computed tomogram remains one of the most expensive pieces of equipment in the department of diagnostic radiology, it follows that the distribution of the basic principals and of applications and limitations of computed tomography among these non-neuroradiologists will increase its cost effectiveness, and more importantly, its proper use.

The book is systematically divided into 10 chapters with the text limited to essentials. Illustrated images with a wide range of quality have purposely been chosen to accurately represent the daily work of a large general hospital. A sufficient number of images from the latest generation models have also been included to allow for reader comparison. This manual is intended to be an introductory text, but for those who are interested in more complete information, an up-to-date bibliography has been appended to each chapter.

New York City   K.Y.C.
                                                       N.F.

Chapter I

Early civilizations believed that the entire world was composed of four elements: fire, air, earth, and water. We now know there are 92 elements. And, ever since Röntgen discovered the X-ray in 1895, radiologists have believed the roentgenogram could display only four components of the human body: gas, bone, fat, and soft tissues. Invasion of the body with contrast materials was necessary to show structure within homogeneous soft tissues.

The advent of computerized tomography has revolutionized radiology. A mathematic reconstruction from a series of transmitted X-ray beams through the body allows this new radiologic modality to differentiate various types of tissues—including abscesses, neoplasms, and cysts—heretofore invisible in the intact body.

The conventional radiograph is not able to differentiate linear attenuations much less than 5 percent. At least three factors limit our ability to detect tissue differences in soft tissue areas. These are: (a) the presence of scattered radiation from the patient; (b) the inability of the film-screen system to record differences less than 2 percent in X-ray transmission; and (c) loss of information because three-dimensional data have been superimposed on a two-dimensional imaging system.

On the other hand, the computerized tomograph can distinguish linear attenuations as low as 0.5 percent (fig. 1). This improvement is so dramatic and diagnostically revealing, it held a secure and unquestioned position in our diagnostic armamentarium 3 years after it became available.

Conventional Radiography

Exposure of a conventional radiograph involves a beam of X-rays that pass through the body, where it is differentially attenuated by various tissues. It then impinges on a film-screen system, the image detector. The same principle applies when the image detector is a fluorescent screen, an image intensifier tube, or a selenium coated plate (xerography).

In the case of the film-screen, the X-ray beam interacts with the screen, producing light that exposes the film. The film is developed to produce an image. In areas of the body where attenuation is high (bone), very few X-ray photons reach the film and the resultant image is white or clear. In areas where there is little attenuation (lung), many X-ray photons pass through the object, and the resultant image is black or dark.

Attenuation is a function of several variables and processes. Generally, the degree of attenuation increases with increased physical density, increased thickness, and an increased atomic number of the attenuator. It decreases with increasing X-ray photon energy. Hence, on a radiograph, fat with a low atomic number and density will appear rela-

Principles of Computerized Axial Tomography

1A

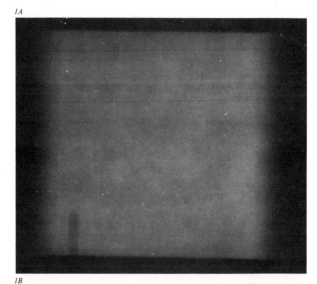

1B

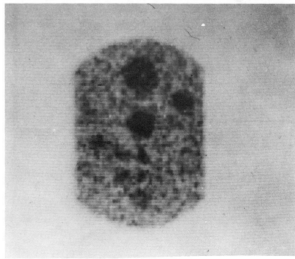

Fig. 1. Phantom consists of polycarbonate plastic rods in nylon. There is a 1% difference in attenuation between the two plastic materials.
A Roentgenogram does not visualize rods.
B CT scan visualizes many rods of various diameters.

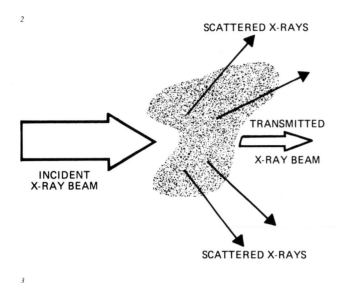

Fig. 2. Attenuation of X-rays passing through matter results in fewer photons remaining in original path. Scattered photons may degrade the final image (courtesy of General Electric Company).

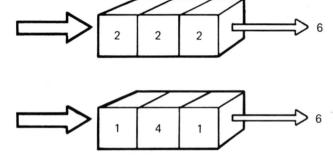

Fig. 3. Combinations of different structures, with different radiation attenuation values, can result in similar total attenuations, thus producing images that look the same (courtesy of General Electric Company).

tively dark due to low attenuation, whereas bone, which has a higher density and atomic number, will appear light, indicating greater attenuation.

Attenuation is a result of either of two separate interactions between an X-ray photon and the atoms of the material through which it is passing (fig. 2). *Photoelectric absorption* is the result of photon interaction with the inner electrons of an atom so that the entire energy of the photon is transferred to an electron and the photon disappears. *Compton scattering* occurs when an X-ray photon interacts with the orbital electron of an atom with only partial transfer or energy. This photon remains in existence but has reduced energy and, more important, it changes direction; it has been scattered.

A roentgenogram is, in effect, a shadowgram produced by X-rays passing through the body. The beams that pass directly from the source to the film without undergoing Compton scattering carry the significant information. Photons that reach the film after undergoing Compton scattering no longer maintain a true geometric relationship and act as *noise* in the image, adding to the exposure without increasing information content. The result is a degradation of image quality, especially in contrast and detail.

The individual X-ray, which reaches any point on a radiograph, has been influenced by multiple processes that degrade the final image. Each element of tissue through which it has passed has attenuated it to some degree. The final information it carries is the sum of the individual attenuations of each piece of matter through which it has passed. This means that different combinations of attenuations can result in similar information being transmitted by the primary beam to the film (fig. 3).

It is obvious, but worthy of emphasis, that a radiograph is a two-dimensional film that images a three-dimensional object. The effects of overlapping structures and the small differences in attenuations and scatter result in an inability to see the internal structure of an organ. Thus, the usual roentgenographic film will not allow our eye to differentiate soft tissues, such as blood, urine, muscle, blood vessels, fibrous tissue, abscesses, cysts, and tumors.

Conventional Tomography

One of the problems in conventional radiography is the superimposition of the shadow of one structure on that of another. Conventional tomography is a mechanical manipulation that allows visualization of a slice or plane within the body by blurring-out tissues above and below the area of interest.

The process involves moving the X-ray tube and the film during exposure in a synchronous but complementary manner. All structures within the plane denoted by the axis of this motion cast shadows that are constant on the film and remain in focus. Structures above or below this plane cast shadows that move on the film and are, therefore, blurred. The blurred planes, however, are still present and contribute to the degradation of image quality.

As we shall see, in contrast to computerized tomography, conventional tomography radiates an entire portion of the body to see one plane or slice in focus. Computerized tomography, utilizing special collimation, radiates only a selected plane or slice, and eliminates both unnecessary radiation to areas of the body outside the plane of interest and the blurring inherent in conventional tomography.

Computerized Tomography

The Computerized Tomography Scanner (CT scanner) is a marriage of conventional X-ray equipment with modern computers. The computer works with numbers that reflect the absorption of a beam of X-rays through a specific portion of the body. The computer knows, in any pinpoint linear path through the area of interest, how much X-ray entered and how much left the body. The difference is the amount of attenuation. These data are used by the computerized tomographic unit to generate, display, and record cross-sectional images (slices) of the human body.

The mathematician *Radon* (1917) showed that a two- or three-dimensional object can be reconstructed from the infinite set of all its projections. The same mathematic con-

struction has been used by astronomers, electron microscopists, and radiologists. Its use in radiology was first proposed by *Oldendorf* in 1961.

In 1969, *Hounsfield*, an English researcher working for EMI Limited, developed a prototype device based on the reconstruction principle. In collaboration with Dr. J. Ambrose, studies were made of the human brain, and it was demonstrated that a tumor could be differentiated from its surrounding tissue. A clinical prototype was then constructed and installed. Results were presented in April 1972, at the Annual Congress of the British Institute of Radiology.

In the United States, units were installed at the Mayo Clinic and the Massachusetts General Hospital in 1973. Results were reported early in 1974 with enthusiastic responses.

The first EMI Scanner was limited to head scanning. A different device capable of scanning the body was developed and put into operation by *R.S. Ledley* at Georgetown University in early 1974. This was commercially developed as the ACTA Scanner; the first model was installed at the University of Minnesota Hospital in 1975. Almost concurrently, the Technicare Corporation developed a body scanner called the Delta Scanner, which was installed in the Cleveland Clinic as a prototype in the Spring of 1975 and as a commercial model at the New England Medical Center in July 1975.

The original EMI device could only scan the brain and took 5 minutes to scan a single slice. Recent machines are able to scan any portion of the body at speeds as fast as 1 second.

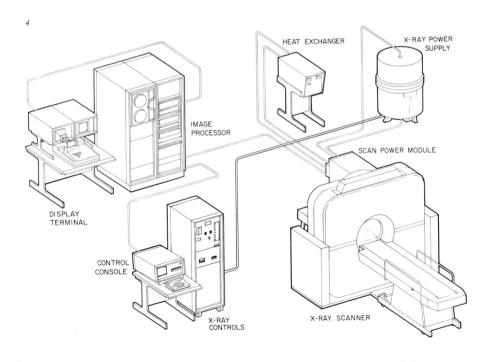

Fig. 4. Components of a CT system. X-ray scanner consists of gantry and motorized patient table. Image processor is the computer and images are seen and photographed at the display terminal (courtesy of Technicare Corporation).

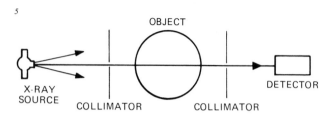

5

OBJECT

X-RAY
SOURCE

COLLIMATOR

COLLIMATOR

DETECTOR

Fig. 5. Production of a finely collimated X-ray beam.

CT Equipment

A typical CT device is composed of a scanning gantry, (fig. 4) containing the X-ray source, radiation detectors, and measuring electronics; a scanning table; X-ray power supply and controls; a computer; and viewing devices (fig. 5). Some units also contain a heat exchanger to help dissipate the heat generated in the X-ray tube.

The X-ray source is either a fixed or rotating anode X-ray tube. In general, the translate-rotate machines use a fixed anode therapy type X-ray tube, which is operational during the entire scan. Newer designs use a diagnostic type rotating anode tube and may pulse the X-ray beam on and off during the scan.

The detectors that convert the transmitted X-ray intensity into an electric signal have been both scintillation crystal and gas types. Scintillators have been sodium iodide (NaI), calcium fluoride (CaF_2), cesium iodide (CsI), and bismuth germinate (BiGeO). These are coupled to photomultiplier tubes or solid state photodiodes. Gas detectors have been of pressurized Xenon assembled to contain many small ionization chambers.

A special table supports the patient during head and body scanning. It generally is automatically incremented in-and-out and up-and-down to provide precise patient location for multiple scans. Some of the less expensive machines have manual incrementing. The X-ray power supply ranges from simple to complex; single phase units through constant potential devices have been used.

Computers have been of the small dedicated type. The computer size, peripheral equipment, and hard wired computation boards depend on the matrix size used, the speed of reconstruction required, and the reconstruction algorithm.

Viewing devices are usually television or cathode-ray tubes. These devices display images either in shades of gray or in color, and can be adjusted to control contrast, latitude, and numerical region of interest.

Permanent images are obtained by photographing the primary display or a secondary (slave) screen, using conventional or Polaroid films. Multiple images, on X-ray film, can be made using special slave imager cameras. The images and data can be permanently stored on film or by digital recording on magnetic tape or discs.

Computer Data Collection

The theory of image reconstruction is based on the concept that the internal structure of an object can be derived from a series of transmission measurements made by probing the object from all angles, with many finely collimated X-ray beams. The transmission measurement is the difference between an entrance beam of known intensity and the output intensity after the beam has passed through the body. These transmission measurements can be used to mathematically reconstruct the internal structure. The more angles (views) measured and the more transmission measurements taken per view, the more accurately the reconstruction represents the scanned object. There are two steps to the generation of a CT scan slice—data acquisition and mathematic reconstruction—which can be performed either sequentially or simultaneously, depending on the manufacturer's choice of design.

The objective of the *data acquisition phase* is to obtain a series of X-ray projections from several angles, through the object being scanned. Each projection is a series of individual, highly collimated X-ray transmission measurements taken across the designated plane in each patient. Early machines used a process called translate-rotate for this purpose. In this process, a highly collimated pencil beam of X-rays (fig. 5) was passed through the object being scanned. The beam was then detected by a sensitive X-ray detector system, such as a sodium iodide crystal and photomultiplier tube. The earliest machine had only one pair of detectors; later designs had six and up to 30. These allowed faster scans, and in some cases gathered data for two adjacent slices simultaneously. There was also another detector on the input side, so that actual absorption measurements could be determined by subtracting the output from the input intensity.

The X-ray source and detector assembly are traversed across the subject being scanned (fig. 6), while a number of individual transmission measurements are made. The entire assembly is then rotated a predetermined amount (fig. 7)—usually 1° for a single detector system and more for multiple detector systems where multiple angle data are gathered simultaneously (fig. 8)—and another traverse initiated. This is continued until 180° have been covered, thus ensuring that every element in the object is viewed from every angle.

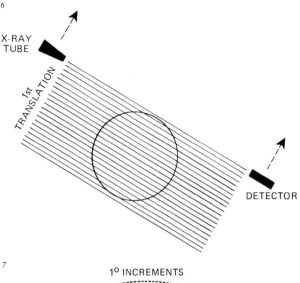

6

Fig. 6. Diagram of first translation of a translate-rotate CT machine (courtesy of General Electric Company).

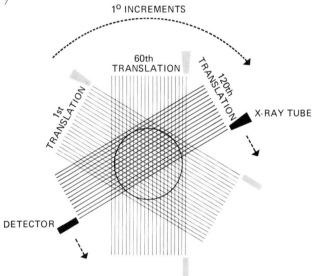

7

Fig. 7. Scanning motions of a first generation (translate-rotate) CT scanner (courtesy of General Electric Company).

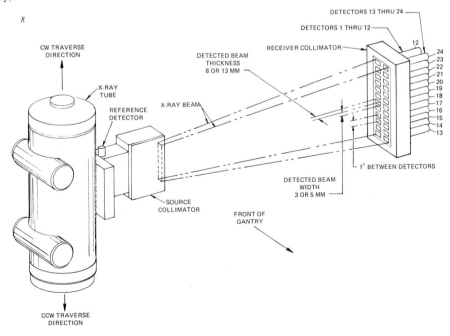

8

Fig. 8. Diagram of a multiple detector CT Scanner of translate-rotate type. Multiple detectors allow scanning speeds as fast as 18 sec/slice (courtesy of Technicare Corporation).

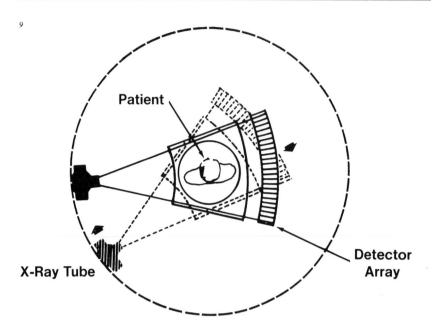

Fig. 9. A typical third generation CT Scanner. The thin but wide fan beam covers the entire patient "slice" and rotates with the detector usually over 360°.

For each traverse, several thousand X-ray transmission measurements enter the computer.

When a scan is completed, the patient is moved a preselected distance and another scan-slice procedure started. This process is continued until the number of slices necessary for a complete study of the area of interest has been done. The thickness of the slice is nominally the thickness of the X-ray beam, which is controlled by collimation at the source and at the detector. This thickness generally ranges from 3 to 15 mm. Motion is an important source of error in the reconstruction, especially in scans of the chest or abdomen. Scan time is, therefore, an important consideration. The time necessary to gather the data for a slice reconstruction has been reduced by adding detectors and increasing the speed of translation and rotation. The fastest scan done by a translate-rotate type machine is completed in about 10 seconds.

The newest designs have replaced translate-rotate motion with a continuous circular motion over 360°. Two different detector approaches have been used. Both rely on a fan-shaped X-ray beam that passes through the entire body slice being scanned at all times. The first type uses a multiple array of detectors that rotate opposite to the X-ray source. The detector is an assembly of many small gas-filled ionization chambers. The second type uses many stationary detectors located in a circular array, with only the source rotating. These designs have reduced the time necessary for a single scan to the order of 1 second.

Generations of CT Scanners

Since the introduction of EMI Head Scanner, there has been a rapid explosion in the technology of CT scanners, with the following goals: the ability to scan the body as well as the head, faster scanning speed, faster reconstruction time, improved accuracy of reconstruction, and better resolution.

The industry has tended to describe these changes by designating the more significant advances as different generations. Generally, the designation of a new generation has indicated a new design in scanning geometry. This generalizing has tended to cloud the distinction between machines within a given "generation." In fact, various manufacturers have chosen to emphasize and improve different aspects of their machines. These changes, whether due to specific expertise, the inventiveness of a particular engineering department, the availability of a particular technology, cost, or for some marketing advantage, have resulted in significant differences between the machines of different manufacturers within the same "generation."

Using the definitions generally used in the industry, *the first generation* has the original EMI and ACTA machines as its examples. These machines use a single, pencil-beam X-ray source and a single detector. Motion is of the translate-rotate design. A single slice requires 4 to 5 minutes of scan time and a similar amount of reconstruction time.

The second generation of machines are of two types (2A and 2B), both of which still use the translate-rotate motion for scanning. However, by using multiple detectors and collimating the X-ray source into several beams, information can be collected at a faster rate (fig. 9). This results in decreased scanning time. Improvement in the computer and calculation process also reduces reconstruction time. Most of the machines are also designed so that body sections could be obtained along with those of the head on a single machine.

The 2A generation (an example of which is the Delta 50 machine) was designed with two sets of three detectors so that two adjacent slices can be scanned simultaneously. Scan time is about 2½ minutes, and the image is reconstructed almost immediately after all data have been acquired. The reconstruction of one slice can be viewed as the data are being collected.

The use of multiple detectors was carried further by some manufacturers, resulting in the 2B generation. The machines still use the translate-rotate motion but now have 12 to 30 detectors per slice. The resulting scan time is about 18 seconds (Delta 50 Fast Scan), and in one case 10 seconds (Elscint). Images are available 10 seconds to 3 minutes after the data have been acquired.

The third generation (example General Electric) departs from the first two in that the translate portion of the scan motion is eliminated (fig. 9). The X-ray beam is collimated to form a thin fan intercepted by an arc of detectors that rotate opposite to the source of X-rays. The simpler motion and reduction of vibration allow scan times of about 5 seconds. Reconstruction time is on the order of 1 minute.

The fourth generation (Pfizer, Picker, Technicare) started when the speed of scanning was increased by rotating only the tube. The detectors do not move but are arranged in a 360° array. The moving X-ray source with a fan beam effectively uses up to 720 individual detectors in this design.

The third and fourth generation scanners are equal in speed and in the excellent quality of their diagnostic images. Detail is excellent, and motion artifacts are reduced to a minimum.

Formation of the Image

Since the computer deals only with numbers (absorption at individual points), it is necessary to change the numbers for each point (pixel) in the body slice to a shade of white, gray, or black (or color) to get an image. Let us see how this is accomplished.

The reconstruction phase of the scan is that phase during which the various transmission measurements are used to reconstruct an image representative of the "slice" of body being scanned. This begins with the determination of numbers (digitally) and is accomplished by the scan computer, or in most cases a specially wired computation board. The recipe used to perform the reconstruction is called an algorithm. The result of the reconstruction is a group of numbers called a matrix. A matrix is defined as an array of numbers arranged in rows and columns; each individual number is an element of the matrix. Matrix sizes commonly used in computed tomography are 128×128, 160×160, 256×256, 320×320, and 512×512, each number representing

one point in the matrix. These points are called *pixels,* which means picture element. Each pixel corresponds to a geometrically equivalent volume element (*voxel*) in the original object scanned. A machine that used a 256×256 matrix would have 64,536 elements, but since the scanning procedure describes a circle, the corners are not calculated. The result is only 50,660 points (pixels). Fewer data points result in a faster computation and image production.

The CT reconstruction assigns each pixel a number related to the average linear attenuation coefficient for the volume (voxel) element corresponding to that point. There are several algebraic methods for obtaining these numbers.

The problem can be illustrated by a simple puzzle. Image a square that has been divided into four small boxes. Each of these small boxes contains a number, which is unknown. All that is known is the sum for each of the two rows and the two columns. You are to determine the numbers in the four boxes. A problem of this magnitude could probably be done mentally; or you might resort to a simple trial-and-error process. In the latter instance, you would guess at your answer, see if it satisfied the row and column sums, then make corrections to improve your guess. This would continue several times until you solved the problem. Now imagine what would happen to your solution process if the square was 3×3, then 4×4, then 5×5, and so on. Very quickly, the problem would surpass either your capability or time. To solve a matrix of 256×256 pixels, several million calculations would be necessary; the solution of this type of problem in a reasonable period of time is made possible by a digital computer.

There are several approaches to the described type of problem. The simplest is a method similar to the trial and error described for the simple puzzle above. The process is called *iteration,* whereby a series of successive approximations are made, starting with an arbitrary value for each pixel. Between each approximation, correction terms are developed from the error between the pixel sums and the actual measured projection values. These corrections are applied to the pixel values and the process starts again. When the error is sufficiently small, the process is stopped, and the resulting pixel values for attenuation are a close approximation to the actual values in the object that has been scanned.

The *back projection method* is a simpler reconstruction procedure. In this process the value of the detected projection signal is divided equally among all pixels comprising that projection value. After the values of all projections have been so divided and added to their respective pixels, an approximation of the original object results. Each pixel is proportional to the sum of all rays projected through it.

This method of reconstruction has an inherent artifact (called the star pattern), which renders it unsuitable for accurate reconstruction of objects. This is because pixels outside an area in the slice are assigned some of the density

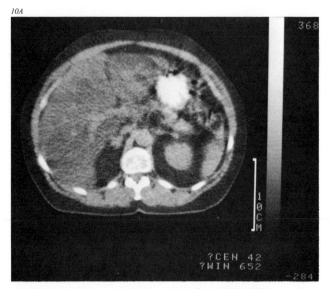

10A

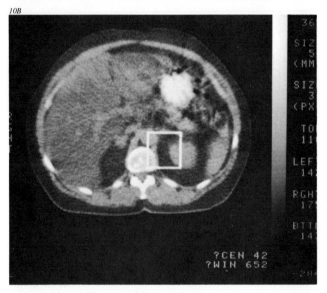

10B

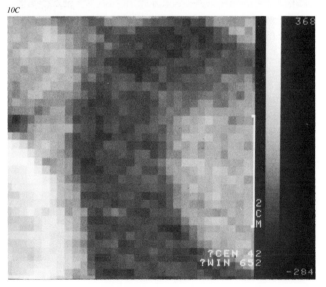

10C

value associated with the projection of that area. The practical result of this method of reconstruction is that detail in the image is blurred.

The analytic method commonly used for reconstruction is based on a modified back-projection concept, known as *filtered-back projection* or convolution. The process is similar to the back-projection method with an extra step: at the end of each projection, the transmission values are modified by the application of a filter function before apportionment to the pixels. The filter has the effect of compensating for the blurring caused by the star effect. The choice of filter function will affect the clarity of the resulting image and the presence or absence of some types of artifacts.

This method offers the advantage of allowing reconstruction to proceed simultaneously with the scan. Each projection profile can be processed as soon as it is measured so that the image can be monitored during the scanning process.

Another method is called *fast fourier transform* (FFT). This method takes advantage of the repetitive nature of sine and cosine functions to reduce the number of mathematic manipulations necessary to solve the reconstruction.

The choice of algorithm rests with the designer of the CT device. The objectives are to perform the reconstruction as rapidly as possible, reduce the number of mathematic processes necessary to achieve a solution, optimize resolution of detail, minimize artifacts and distortions, and so on. These goals are not mutually exclusive and much research time and effort is being expended in investigating different methods of reaching a better solution.

The Diagnostic CT Image: Window Width and Window Level

Remember that the solution to the reconstruction problem is a matrix of numbers (fig. 10). Each number is directly related to the average linear attenuation of X-rays in its associated voxel. This is important because the radiologist generally does not look at these numbers; instead, he looks at a picture (fig. 10). This picture must be generated from the information contained in the reconstruction matrix,

Fig. 10. The CT image.

A A typical image of a CT Scan (slice) through the abdomen. There is dilute contrast material in the stomach. Liver is on the right and a portion of the left kidney is seen. Patient is supine. Note that picture indicates certain basic information: right side, center (+42) and limits of window (+368 to −284) and centimeter scale. Indentification of patient, institution and date of examination can also be added via the computer.

B Area outlined by the white rectangle has been selected for enlargement.

C The enlarged area is now imaged. We can now identify the individual pixels with their various shades of gray.

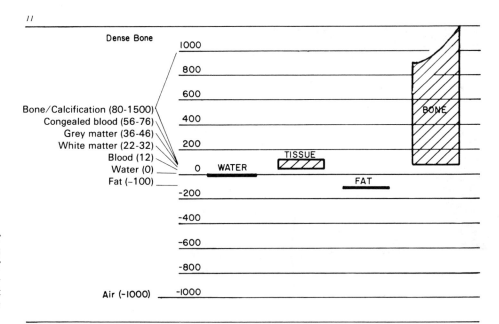

Fig. 11. Graph indicating CT numerical values (Hounsfield units) for various tissues. Since the CT number is related to the linear attenuation coefficient of a tissue, it can be used diagnostically (courtesy of Technicare Corporation).

which requires further processing by the CT system. A basic understanding of this process is necessary, if one is not to be misled by distortions caused by the conversion process.

Generally, the conversion of pixel values to shades of gray will be controlled by two parameters: center and window width. Most CT scanners work on a scale of pixel values that range from −1000 to +1000. Water attenuation is set to be zero. Under this system, most biologic tissue will fall within the range of −50 to +100. Suppose now that the display system operated with 32 shades of gray. The centering control will determine the pixel numbers that will correspond to the sixteenth-shade of gray. The window adjustment will determine the range of extreme values that will correspond to the white and black shades. Both of these parameters can generally be adjusted over the entire range of pixel numbers.

Let us now assume we have set a window of 100 and a center value of plus 50. With this system, any value less than zero will show black and any value greater than 100 will show white. Note that we will not see any detail for biologic tissue with pixel values between 0 and −50; it will all be given the black shade. Since we have 32 shades of gray, each shadow will represent three pixel values.

Suppose now that the center is moved to −150. The shades of gray will represent CT values ranging from −100 to −200. Information in our biologically important range will not be present in the image since its CT values will all be converted to the same white shade.

Return the center to +50 and expand the window to 400. Our range of conversion into shades of gray will now be from −150 to +250, with each shade representing 12 CT numbers. If we are looking for differences in the image,

which are less than 12 CT numbers spart, we will have difficulty, since they will have the same shade of gray.

This example illustrates the use of the display control. Different systems might use different nomenclature or control ranges, but the concept is the same. Figure 11 shows the CT numbers for various types of tissue. Our interest should be centered on the soft tissues, which vary from 0 to +76 in this schema. Differences of 10 to 12 in the CT number (Hounsfield unit) may be important in the differentiation of various types of fluid and soft tissues.

One must also consider the physiology of the eye and the response of the image display device. The eye is not capable of seeing more than 15 shades of gray. Various films have less capacity; they are only able to display eight or 10 shades. The television monitor is not necessarily linear in its ability to convert a voltage level to a shade of gray. If it tends to compress levels, let's say at the white (bright) end of its range, then the ability to use the picture to interpret various CT numbers is further compromised. Understanding these factors will explain some undesired or unexpected images; on the other hand, this knowledge may help the operator to visualize areas of special interest. A special handle or joystick that allows the computer to give an average CT number for an area of interest, is standard equipment on most machines.

Quality Control

Many manufacturers of CT machines provide phantoms that can be used to monitor performance. Some also provide computer programs to complement this function. These de-

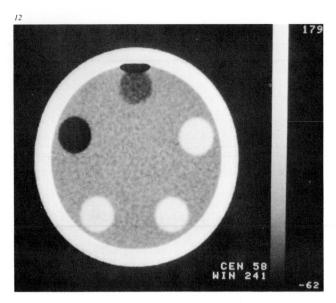

12
179
CEN 58
WIN 241
-62

Fig. 12. Scan of a CT performance phantom. This phantom allows the rapid determination of noise level and contrast linearity. The mottled gray area in the center of the circle is water; the mottling is due to noise. The five small circles are five different plastics with known X-ray absorption properties and therefore predetermined CT values.

vices are quite important because they assure the operator that the machine functions consistently and at peak performance day after day. Although the CT unit provides rather precise information, it is subject to many disturbances that affect its function. The malfunction is not always apparent in the scan, and as a simple test that can be done each day, scan a lucite cylinder filled with water. Since the CT (Hounsfield) number for water generally averages zero, any significant deviation indicates a change in performance.

If the phantom contains small blocks of several different materials (fig. 12), such as plastics, their X-ray absorption properties can be determined independently, and the CT values assigned to them during a scan can then be used to monitor the linearity of the scanner. Many other simple tests are suggested by the manufacturer, or can be devised. Many appear in a monograph on CT quality control published by the American Association of Physicists in Medicine.

Complications

Noise

The interactions of photons with matter is statistical in nature. Therefore, there is always a degree of uncertainty whenever a process related to photon interactions is involved. An example is the quantum mottle in the conventional radiograph. This phenomenon is the increased error caused as fewer photons generate an image when a faster screen or film is used to reduce radiation exposure.

In a CT system, noise results from electronic variation in components, random (statistical) fluctuation of the X-ray beam and the response and uniformity of the detectors, stability of the X-ray power supply, and the quantum nature of the photon-detector interaction. Noise affects the practical use of a CT device. It adds an error factor to any CT number measurement, and it can cause graininess in the viewed image.

Noise can be evaluated by scanning a uniform object (water bath). The distribution of CT numbers will have a standard deviation that can be used to evaluate the noise level. In the image, the noise will manifest itself in the nonuniformity of homogeneous areas.

Various manufacturers have approached the problem of noise in different ways. The choice of algorithm, patient dose, and design resolution all affect this parameter. It should be an important consideration in choosing CT equipment.

Motion

Motion is perhaps the most common artifact in a CT reconstruction. This is due to the fact that the body is a dynamic object and a scan takes a definite time to perform. The mathematic solution assumes that the several projections that comprise the reconstruction are all of the same object slice. When motion occurs, this is no longer true, and the result is loss of resolution and streak artifacts. Therefore, the patient as well as the developing image should be observed during the study. If motion occurs, the diagnostic quality of the image can be evaluated immediately, and the scan aborted or repeated, if necessary. The motion artifact has been a prime reason for the development of faster scanners. The 2-minute machines were adequate for head work, but respiration, peristalsis, and patient motion greatly limited their use for body work.

X-ray Spectra

If the X-ray beam in a CT scanner were monoenergetic, this complication would not exist. Unfortunately, the beam is composed of a spectrum of energies, and its attenuation in matter is a function of energy. As higher energy photons are less strongly attenuated, a higher percentage of the lower energy photons are selectively removed from the beam as it passes through the body. As a result, the attenuation coefficient is not a constant but a function of the material thickness. The CT value of a pixel, then, is related to its relative position in the body. This must be corrected in the reconstruction process. The early EMI Scanner used a water bag, so that the X-ray beam always passed through a constant thickness of material. This limited the scanner to head work only.

Later machines tried software correction in the computer by developing a correction factor determined from a scan of homogeneous material. Others resorted to an external bolus material to approximate a cylinder, or used compensating filters in the beam. A combination of these methods are now being used by some manufacturers.

Other Artifacts

Several other artifacts are commonly encountered. As a radiologist becomes familiar with a machine, he or she will begin to recognize and discount them.

Strong absorbents, such as tooth fillings or contrast material, can have absorption that exceeds the machine's ability to accurately digitize their effect on transmission. The result is a distortion error, which is introduced by the scan data. On the image, this might appear as an inappropriate CT value or gray-shade inversion. This results from the de-

sign of a digital counter, which, after reaching its limits, starts over at zero. Another manifestation of this type of absorber is a streak artifact that radiates from the abnormal material in the image.

Strong absorbers such as bone produce another type of artifact. This is a result of two effects: (a) an interpolation during calculation, which cannot account for the rapid change in attenuation factors, and (b) a failure in the beam-hardening correction (fig. 13), which is an average correction. The result is broad streaking of reduced CT numbers, extending from the strong absorber on the image. On a head scan, the reduced CT numbers, which appear between the image of the petrous ridges, is an example of this artifact.

The original EMI machine had an overshoot that appeared next to a strong-weak absorber interface. It was originally thought that this was a visualization of the subarachnoid space, but we now know it is an artifact produced by the reconstruction algorithm. In newer machines, this same artifact is related to the choice of filter function, which can be designed to give very sharp boundaries (fig. 14) within the image. If the requirement for sharpness is relaxed, the artifact can be eliminated.

Some of the newer designs offer a choice of solution algorithms to the operator. A choice can then be made, based on clinical needs, as to what compromises should be made concerning sharpness and artifacts.

Room Design

Proper planning, during the design of the environment for a CT machine, will reduce the incidence of problems

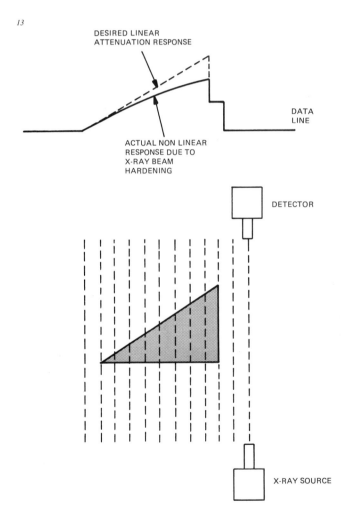

Fig. 13. Diagram of the effect of the beam hardening artifact. A heterogeneous beam of X-rays is hardened when passing through increasing thickness of absorber because the lower energy X-rays are selectively absorbed.

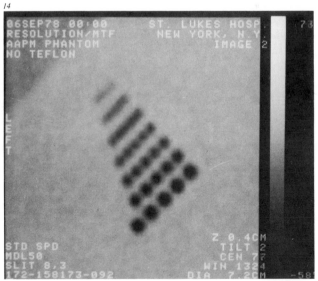

Fig. 14. Phantom to evaluate resolution. This image is a scan of a plastic cylinder with a series of progressively smaller holes; the center row of holes are 1.5 mm in diameter.

during its operation. Computers, disc drives, heat exchangers, and other such parts are not commonly found in a radiology department. Past experience, therefore, may not be available, and one must rely on outside support for design assistance. These devices need an environment in which temperature, humidity, and dust levels are controlled much more rigorously than in the usual X-ray suite.

Transistors, when they become warm, can malfunction. In a computer, this leads to erroneous results and sometimes complete failure. Air-conditioning requirements must, therefore, be considered in the design. This should include the effect on people working in the room plus the heat-load generated by the equipment. In many installations this will mean the addition of auxiliary air-conditioning, which should probably be oversized to allow for aging. Contingency plans for machine operation should also be made in the event that this auxiliary unit fails. The alternative is to shut the machine down until it is required.

Humidity can be either too high or too low. High humidity accelerates the breakdown of electronic components (capacitors, switches, and others), thereby increasing machine down-time. Low humidity will allow the buildup of static. This generally leads to spurious signals in the computer system, which are guaranteed to happen at the most inopportune time.

The head of a disc drive rides only several microns above the disc. This distance is much less than the diameter of a human hair. Therefore, dust control is very important, because dust acts as an abrasive and will eventually cause data loss or distortion. A large particle can even cause the drive to "crash" so that the disc must be replaced and the drive mechanism repaired.

Dust and environmental control should extend beyond the normal working hours. In one instance, extensive machine down-time was found to be caused by housekeeping. Iron particles from a steel-wool pad that had been used to clean the floors entered the computer and were causing random shorts.

In allocating space, consideration should be given to adequate working room, a patient waiting area, and data storage. The possibility of future expansion needs should be considered.

Radiation Dose

It has always been an axiom in radiology that the ratio between diagnostic information and radiation dose to the patient be maximized. This is because exposure to ionizing radiation is not a benign process.

The same rule applies to CT scanning. Different machines present different amounts of diagnostic information and expose the patient to different doses of radiation. An increased dose, however, does not always mean increased diagnostic information.

A particular machine might be operated in several different modes (usually slower speeds) to improve diagnostic information. When the scan takes longer, the patient dose is increased. Is this additional information worth the increased exposure? Does this machine or procedure balance the lowest radiation dose against the most significant diagnostic information? If these questions are considered, radiologists will usually utilize ionizing radiation wisely.

The clinician often asks: "How does radiation exposure from a CT scan compare to that from some other radiographic study?" This question does not have a simple answer. In a conventional radiograph, a broad beam of radiation impinges upon the patient. It is, therefore, relatively easy to measure the maximum skin dose and estimate or-

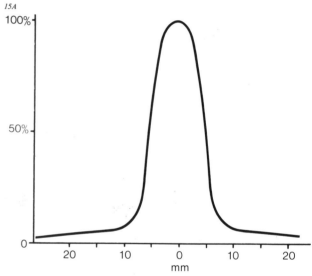

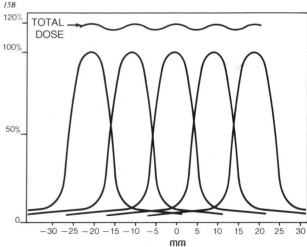

Fig. 15. Dose profiles of CT examinations.
A Axial projection, single slice dose profile.
B Multiple slice dose profile (courtesy of General Electric Company).

gan, bone marrow, and gonadal doses from direct and scattered radiation.

The geometry of a CT machine is different. A very thin, collimated beam or a fan beam is moved around the patient, either 180° or 360°. Single or multiple slices, overlapping or spacing of slices, and the efficiency of collimation are all factors that affect the ''radiation dose.''

Some basic principles should be understood. The dose profile of the X-ray beam in the axial direction is generally shaped like a normal distribution (fig. 15). The manufacturer will employ collimation to utilize as much of the beam width as possible. Nevertheless, there is always some spillover to tissue outside the slice. If more than one slice is taken and the slices are adjacent, then the maximum dose will be higher than for a single slice (fig. 15), since the dose profiles will overlap. If slices are overlapped, the maximum dose will be increased substantially.

In general, if collimation is proper, radiation dosage to the patient is comparable or somewhat greater than that from a standard roentgenographic study of the part under examination.

State of the Art

During the past 5 years, there have been a large number of improvements in computerized tomography equipment. These have resulted in faster scan times, rapid reconstruction for viewing the image almost instantaneously, and improved resolution, including the ability to reconstruct a small portion of the total image on the entire matrix from the raw data.

The X-ray component of the unit has been upgraded with more dedicated X-ray tubes of higher heat tolerance. The third generation X-ray tubes must pulse, and in all instances the X-ray tube is vulnerable, usually requiring two to three new tubes per year, depending on volume and usage. The detectors are also undergoing improvements with a tendency to the utilization of solid-state detectors (without the use of gas or photomultiplier tubes). There is still disagreement about the best detector system and its geometric configuration (so-called third and fourth generation).

Other developments are occurring in the computer hardware (the actual physical devices that do the work of the computer, such as transistors, integrated circuits, discs, tape recorders, and so on) and software (the algorithms or instructions stored in the computer memory that program the computer to perform various functions or solve problems).

Such improvements have allowed many manipulations of the image, resulting in X-ray views of the area to be studied (scout films) that can then be programmed to allow thin slices at proper angles to accurately visualize the area of interest.

Rapid sequencing of images in one or multiple planes allows ''dynamic imaging'' or visualization of the flow of contrast media through the blood vessels in an area of interest.

Measurement of volume, magnification, precise localization for needle puncture and subtraction of the basic image from an image after contrast are improvements currently being assessed.

Bibliography

Bellon EM, Miraldi FD, Wiesen EJ: Performance evaluation of computed tomography scanners using a phantom model. AJR 132:345, 1979.

Brasch RC, Cann CE: Computed tomographic scanning in children: II. an updated comparison of radiation dose and resolving power of commercial scanners. AJR 138:127, 1982.

Brooks RA, Di Chiro G: Beam hardening in X-ray reconstructive tomography. Physiol Med Biol 21:390, 1976.

Brooks RA, Di Chiro G: Theory of image reconstruction in computed tomography. Radiology 117:561, 1975.

Cormack AM: Early two-dimensional reconstruction (CT scanning) and recent topics stemming from it. J Comput Assist Tomogr 4:648, 1980.

Cormack AM: Representation of a function by its line integrals, with some radiological application. II. J Appl Phys 35:2908, 1964.

Crowther A, DeRosier DJ, Klug A: The reconstruction of a three-dimensional structure from projections and its application to electron microscopy. Proc Roy Soc, London A 317:319, 1970.

Edholm P: Image construction in transverse computer tomography. Acta Radiol (Suppl) 346:21, 1975.

Goitein M: Three-dimensional density reconstruction from a series of two-dimensional projections. Nucl Inst Meth 101:509, 1972.

Goldstein A: Simple buoyancy method for measuring computed tomography phantom material densities. Radiology 128:814, 1978.

Hounsfield G: Computerized transverse axial scanning. Part I: Description of the system. Br J Radiol 46:1016, 1973.

Hounsfield GN: Computed medical imaging. J Comput Assist Tomogr 4:665, 1980.

Johns HE, Battista J, Bronskill MJ, et al: Physics of CT scanners: principles and problems. Int J Radiat Oncol Biol Phys 3:45, 1977.

Joseph PM, Hilal SK, Schulz RA, et al: Clinical and experimental investigation of a smoothed CT reconstruction algorithm. Radiology 134:507, 1980.

Kuhl DE, Edwards RQ: Reorganizing data from the transverse section scans of the brain using processing. Radiology 91:975, 1968.

Latchaw RE, Payne JT, Gold LH: Effective atomic number and electron density as measured with a computed tomography scanner: computation and correlation with brain tumor histology. J Comput Assist Tomogr 2:199, 1978.

Ledley RS, DiChiro G, Lusschop AJ, et al: Computerized transaxial X-ray tomography of the human body. Science 186:207, 1974.

Maue-Dickson W, Trefler M, Dickson DR: Comparison of dosimetry and image quality in computed and conventional tomography. Radiology 131:511, 1979.

McCullough EC: Factors affecting the use of quantitative information from a CT scanner. Radiology 124:99, 1977.

McCullough EC, Payne JT: patient dosage in computed tomography Radiology 129:457, 1978.

McCullough EC, Payne JT, Baker HL, et al: Performance evaluation and quality assurance of computed tomography scanners, with illustrations from the EMI, ACTA, and Delta scanners. Radiology 120:173, 1976.

McDavid WD, Waggener RG, Sank VJ, et al: Correlating computed tomographic numbers with physical properties and operating kilovoltage. Radiology 123:761, 1977.

Oldendorf WH: Isolated flying spot detection of radiodensity discontinuities displaying the internal structural pattern of a complex object. IRE Trans Bio-Med Elect BME 8:68, 1961.

Radon J: Ueber die Bestimmung von Funktionen durch ihre Integralwerte langs gewisser Mannigfaltigkeiten. Ber Verh Sachs Akad Wiss 69:262, 1917.

Rao PS, Gregg EC: Attenuation of monoenergetic gamma rays in tissues. AJR 123:631, 1965.

Robb RA, Ritman EL: High speed synchronous volume computed tomography of the heart. Radiology 133:655, 1979.

Smith KT, Solomon DC, Wagner SL: Practical and mathematical aspects of the problem of reconstructing objects from radiographs. Bull Am Math Soc 83:1227, 1977.

Ter-Pogossian MM: Computerized cranial tomography: equipment and physics. Semin Roentgenol 12:13, 1977.

Wolpert SM: Appropriate window settings for CT anatomic measurements. Radiology 132:775, 1979.

Zatz LM, Alvarez RE: Inaccuracy in computed tomography: energy dependence of CT values. Radiology 124:91, 1977.

Technique

The CT scanner uses a 256×256 matrix at 130 kV and 30 mA. It takes 2 minutes to perform one scan that reconstructs two contiguous images, 8 mm thick. The range of densities extends from 0 (water reference) to $+1000$ (bone) and -1000 (air) Hounsfield units (HU). The Hounsfield unit (HU) is twice the equivalent EMI number (μ).

Contrast enhancement is achieved by an intravenous bolus injection of 100 ml of Renografin 76 (92 percent meglumine diatrizoate and 8 percent sodium diatrizoate). In children, the dose of contrast medium is limited to 2 ml/lb up to 100 ml.

The gantry can be angled up to a maximum of 20° to either side of the vertical plane. Routine work is performed with the plane of section angled 25° to Reid's baseline (fig. 16). Reid's baseline (RB), or anthropologic basal line, is an infraorbital meatal line. This line joins the infraorbital point to the superior border of the external auditory meatus.

The canthomeatal line (CM) or orbitomeatal line joins the outer canthus of the eye to the center of the external

Technique and Anatomy

auditory meatus. Reid's baseline and the canthomeatal line meet at an angle of about 10°. The 15° canthomeatal angle planes are, therefore, equivalent to the 25° infraorbital angle planes. The degree of the gantry tilt may vary, depending on the clinical situation.

Anatomy

Five representative CT scans have been chosen for a discussion of anatomy. They are presented with corresponding anatomic drawings in figures 17 to 21. Each drawing is accompanied by an insert that indicates the plane of the cut by a dotted line. The cut is 25° to the infraorbital meatal line

16

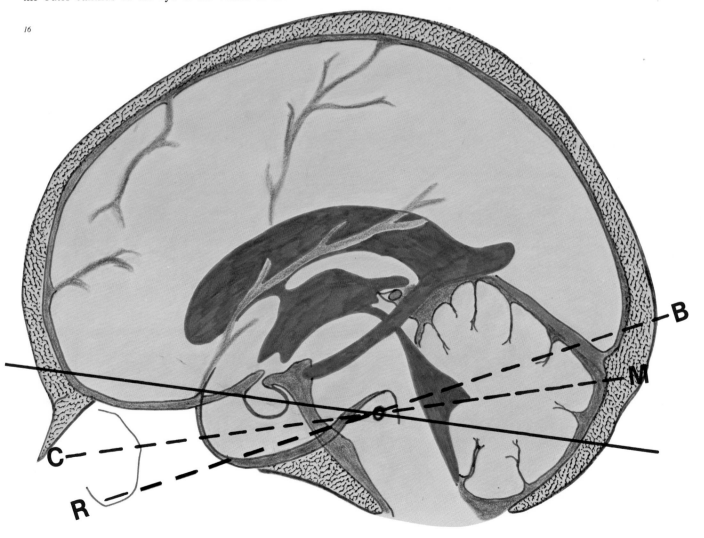

17A

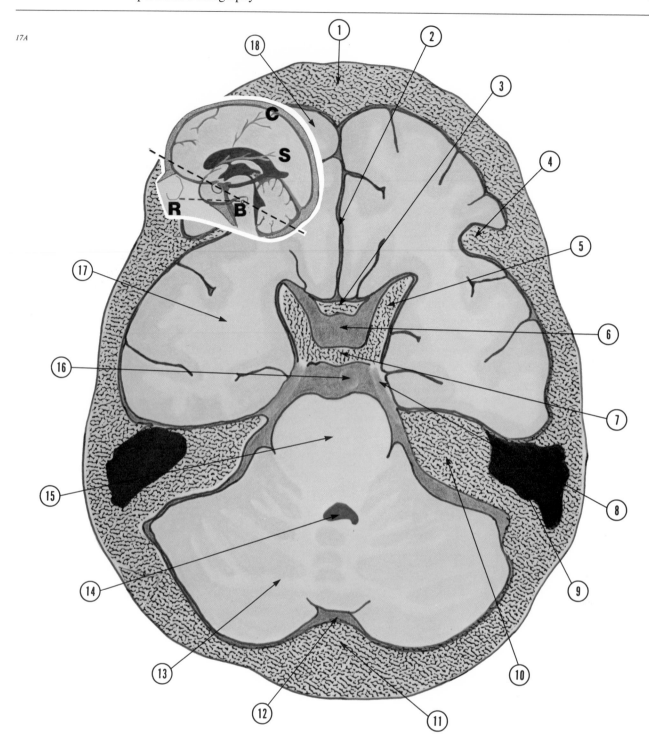

Fig. 17.A.

① frontal bone; ② medial longitudinal fissure and falx cerebri; ③ planum sphenoidale and tuberculum sellae; ④ sphenoid wing; ⑤ anterior clinoid and medial lesser wing; ⑥ suprasellar cistern and pituitary fossa; ⑦ dorsum sellae; ⑧ petroclinoid ligament; ⑨ mastoid sinus; ⑩ petrous pyramid; ⑪ internal occipital protuberance; ⑫ cisterna magna; ⑬ cerebellum; ⑭ IVth ventricle; ⑮ pons; ⑯ basilar artery; ⑰ temporal lobe, inferior part; ⑱ frontal lobe, inferior part.

or Reid's baseline (RB). The sylvian fissure (S) separates the temporal lobe from the parietal lobe, while the central sulcus (C) separates the frontal lobe from the parietal lobe

Bony structures are stippled in black; the ventricular system, basal cisterns, sylvian fissures, and the convolutional sulci are in blue; the enhanced circle of Willis, petroclinoid

Fig. 17.B.

① frontal bone; ② medial longitudinal fissure and falx cerebri; ③ planum sphenoidale and tuberculum sellae; ④ sphenoid wing; ⑤ anterior clinoid and medial lesser wing; ⑥ suprasellar cistern and pituitary fossa; ⑦ dorsum sellae; ⑧ petroclinoid ligament; ⑨ mastoid sinus; ⑩ petrous pyramid; ⑪ internal occipital protuberance; ⑫ cisterna magna; ⑬ cerebellum; ⑭ IVth ventricle; ⑮ pons; ⑯ basilar artery; ⑰ temporal lobe, inferior part; ⑱ frontal lobe, inferior part.

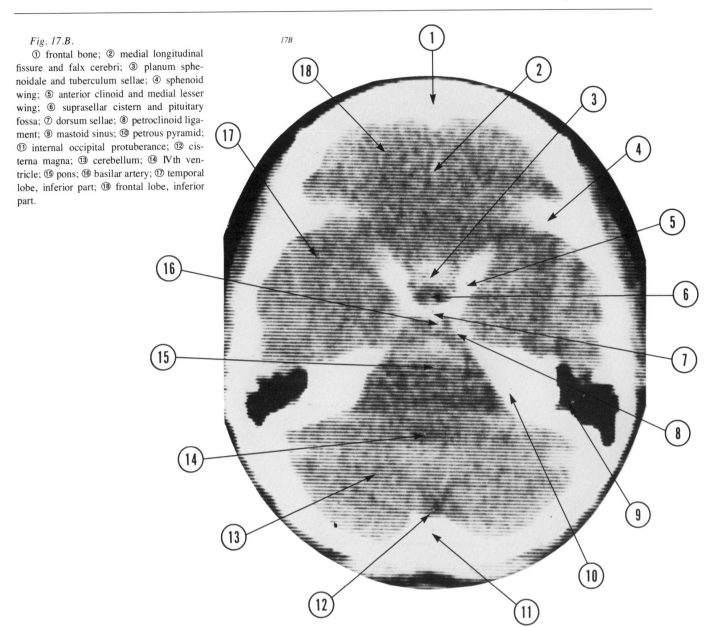

ligaments, falx cerebri, tentorium, the choroid plexus, and the pineal body are in red; and the thalami, caudate nucleus, putamen, and globus pallidus are in brown.

As seen in the insert of figure 17A the scan passes through the interrupted line, which is about 25° to line RB (the Reid's baseline or infraorbitomeatal line). Anteriorly, this scan passes through the inferior portion of the frontal lobe and the temporal lobe, while behind the petrous pyramids it passes obliquely through the pons, the lower fourth ventricle, the inferior vermis, and the lower portion of the cerebellar hemisphere.

On the CT image (fig. 17B) the area of the pons is superimposed by the computer artifacts, with horizontal lucent lines caused by the dense petrous bones and air in the mastoid cells. Even between the left petrous bone and the sphenoid wing, computer artifacts are seen running in the anteroposterior direction. Between the sphenoid wings and the petrous bones, we see the most anterior pole of the temporal lobes.

The bony boundaries of the sella turcica are seen in the center of the scan. Directly anterior to the low density pituitary fossa are the bony tuberculum sellae and planum sphenoidale. Laterally one sees the medial portion of the lesser wing of the sphenoid bone, including the anterior clinoid process. The dorsum sellae is well seen and lies anterior to the enhanced basilar artery.

Anteriorly, the cut passes through the inferior portion of the frontal lobe, just missing the irregular bony orbital roof.

18A

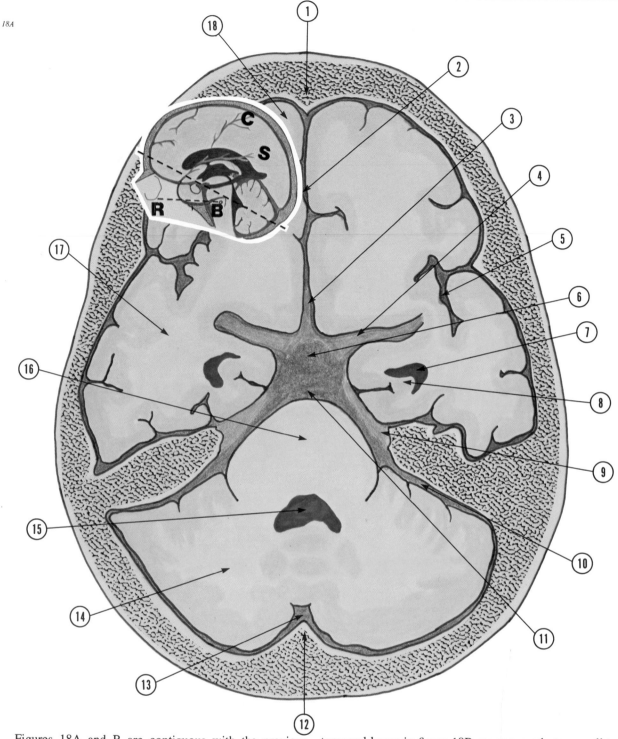

Figures 18A and B are contiguous with the previous scan. Notice the marked difference in the appearance of the sellar area. While the previous lower section predominantly reveals the bony boundaries of the sella turcica, here one sees the suprasellar cistern, the interpenduncular cistern with the basilar artery, and the sylvian fissures with the middle cerebral arteries.

As illustrated by the insert of figure 18A, the scan passes through the most anterior portion of the temporal horns. The

temporal horns in figure 18B are apparently too small to be visualized. But, on another scan (fig. 18C) with a similar scan angle, both temporal horns are well seen (*large arrows*). Here an excellent five-pointed, star-shaped suprasellar cistern can be seen: the longitudinal fissure passes forward in the midline, the sylvian fissures pass anterolaterally on both sides, and the interpeduncular cistern passes posteriorly, within which the basilar artery lies (B). Anteriorly, the scan of figure 18C passes through the lateral part

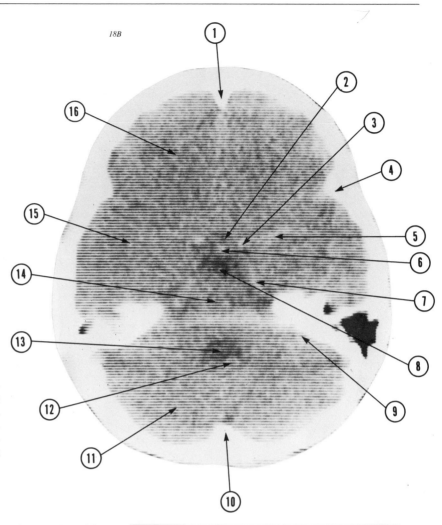

18B

Fig. 18.B.
① Frontal crest; ② suprasellar cistern; ③ carotid siphon, supraclinoid; ④ sphenoid wing; ⑤ middle cerebral artery; ⑥ basilar artery; ⑦ petroclinoid ligament; ⑧ interpeduncular cistern; ⑨ cerebellopontine angle; ⑩ internal occipital protuberance; ⑪ cerebellum; ⑫ choroid plexus; ⑬ IVth ventricle; ⑭ pons; ⑮ temporal lobe; ⑯ frontal lobe.

of the bony orbital roof (the lesser wing of the sphenoid bone and the horizontal portion of the frontal bone), and its plane is, therefore, slightly lower than that of figure 18B.

Posteriorly, this scan passes through the most important landmark of the posterior fossa, namely the fourth ventricle (Figs. 18A–C).

Figures 19A and B are scans through the frontal and temporal lobes, which are separated by the sylvian fissure. The scan is generally not high enough to pass through the central sulcus (C on insert of fig. 19A). Thus, no parietal lobe is included.

The scan passes anteriorly through the frontal horns, in the middle through the oblique plane of the third ventricle, and posteriorly through the upper portions of both leaves of

Fig. 18.A.
① Frontal crest; ② medial longitudinal fissure; ③ anterior cerebral artery; ④ middle cerebral artery; ⑤ sylvian fissure; ⑥ suprasellar cistern; ⑦ temporal horn; ⑧ hippocampus; ⑨ pretroclinoid ligament; ⑩ cerebellopontine angle; ⑪ interpeduncular cistern; ⑫ internal occipital protuberance; ⑬ cisterna magna; ⑭ cerebellum; ⑮ IVth ventricle; ⑯ pons; ⑰ temporal lobe; ⑱ frontal lobe.

19A

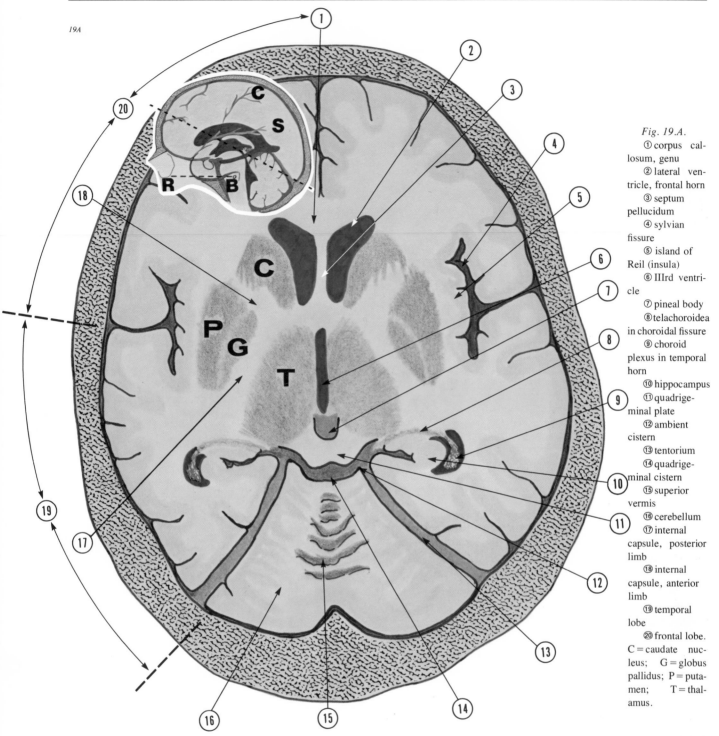

Fig. 19.A.
① corpus callosum, genu
② lateral ventricle, frontal horn
③ septum pellucidum
④ sylvian fissure
⑤ island of Reil (insula)
⑥ IIIrd ventricle
⑦ pineal body
⑧ telachoroidea in choroidal fissure
⑨ choroid plexus in temporal horn
⑩ hippocampus
⑪ quadrigeminal plate
⑫ ambient cistern
⑬ tentorium
⑭ quadrigeminal cistern
⑮ superior vermis
⑯ cerebellum
⑰ internal capsule, posterior limb
⑱ internal capsule, anterior limb
⑲ temporal lobe
⑳ frontal lobe.
C = caudate nucleus; G = globus pallidus; P = putamen; T = thalamus.

the tentorium and the superior vermis and cerebellar hemispheres. On the CT scan (fig. 19B) the quadrigeminal cistern and the enhanced tentorial leaves (*arrows*) delineate the portion of posterior fossa structures included in this scan.

The plane of the scan extends through all basal ganglia; namely, the caudate nucleus (C) and the lentiform nucleus (L) consisting of the putamen (P) and globus pallidus (G). Both thalami (T) are situated lateral to the third ventricle.

Depending on the scan angulation, the level of the ten-

torial leaves traversed by the scan, and the degree of their divergence the appearance of the scan may be quite different posteriorly. In figure 19C, the Gothic arch tentorial blush (*arrows*) is unusually prominent, but normal. The blush corresponds to the tentorial leaves within which the superior vermis lies (V). The anterior end is that part of the tentorial notch through which the scan passes. The linear blush of the falx (*arrowheads*) is very short, indicating that the scan is just above the torcular.

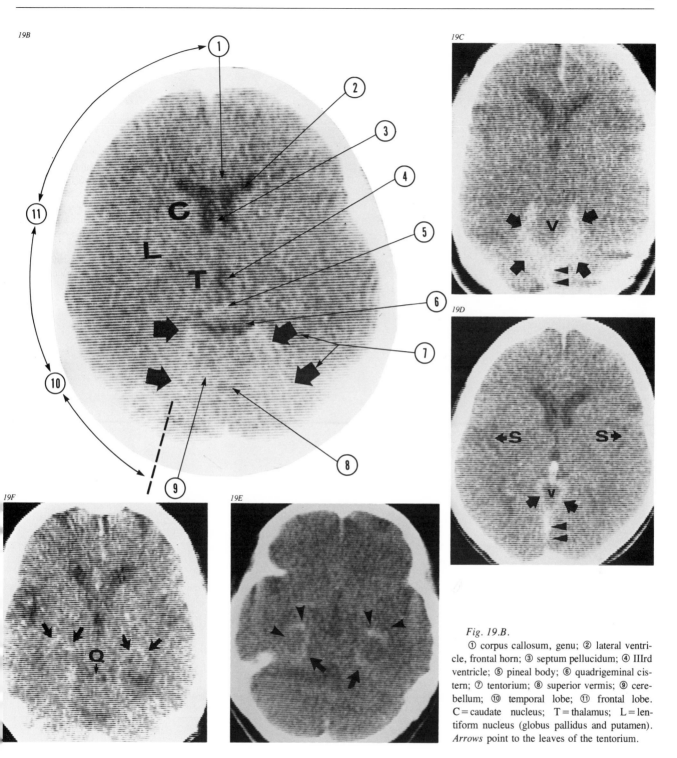

Fig. 19.B.

① corpus callosum, genu; ② lateral ventricle, frontal horn; ③ septum pellucidum; ④ IIIrd ventricle; ⑤ pineal body; ⑥ quadrigeminal cistern; ⑦ tentorium; ⑧ superior vermis; ⑨ cerebellum; ⑩ temporal lobe; ⑪ frontal lobe. C = caudate nucleus; T = thalamus; L = lentiform nucleus (globus pallidus and putamen). *Arrows* point to the leaves of the tentorium.

In figure 19D the scan passes through the tentorial leaves near its apex (*arrows*). The section also passes through a significant portion of the opacified falx (*arrowheads*). The tentorial leaves together with the falx form the Y configuration. The uppermost vermis (V) is situated between the tentorial leaves. The sylvian fissures (A), well seen on both sides, separate the frontal and temporal lobes. Another scan (fig. 19E) taken at a similar angle shows an enhanced tela choroidea in the choroidal fissure, which appears as a thin crescentic density (arrows) extending from the quadrigeminal cistern (Q) to the temporal horn. Figure 19F is an example whereby the choroid plexus of the temporal horn and the enhanced anterior medial edge of the tentorium form an enhanced ring (*arrowheads* and *arrows*). If the head is slightly rotated, and thus only one ring is visible, the finding may be misdiagnosed as a ring-enhanced lesion.

20A

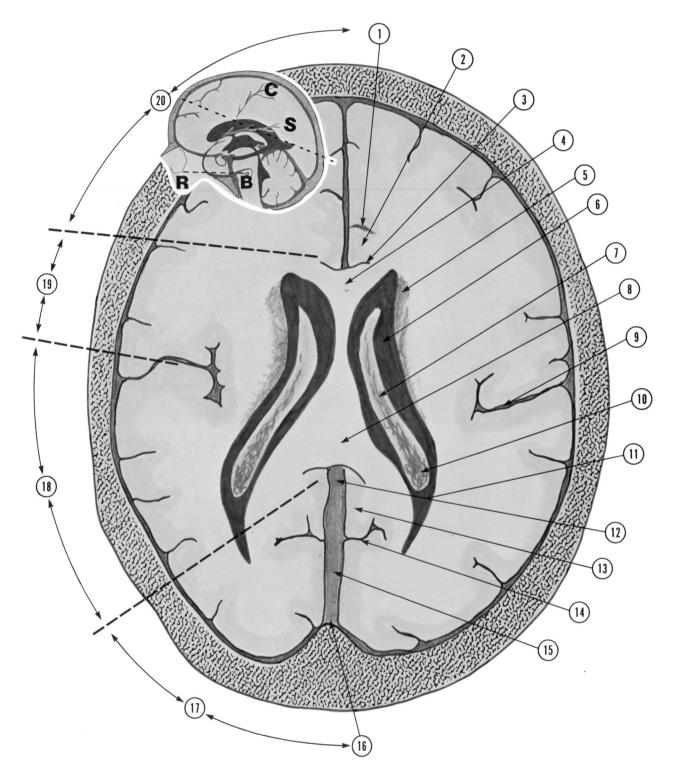

Fig. 20.A.

① cingulate sulcus; ② cingulate gyrus; ③ pericallosal sulcus; ④ corpus callosum, genu; ⑤ caudate nucleus; ⑥ lateral ventricle, body; ⑦ choroid plexus of body of lateral ventricle; ⑧ corpus callosum, splenium; ⑨ sylvian fissure; ⑩ glomus of choroid plexus; ⑪ lateral ventricle, atrium; ⑫ junction of falx and tentorium; ⑬ cingulate gyrus; ⑭ cingulate sulcus; ⑮ posterior falx cerebri; ⑯ superior sagittal sinus; ⑰ occipital lobe; ⑱ temporal lobe; ⑲ parietal lobe; ⑳ frontal lobe.

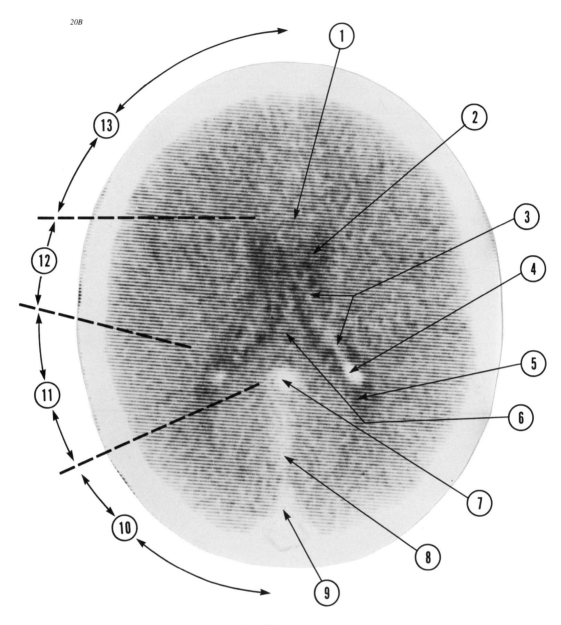

20B

Fig. 20.B.
① corpus callosum, genu; ② lateral ventricle, body; ③ choroid plexus of body of lateral ventricle; ④ glomus of choroid plexus; ⑤ lateral ventricle, atrium; ⑥ corpus callosum, splenium; ⑦ junction of falx and tentorium (vein of Galen); ⑧ posterior falx cerebri; ⑨ superior sagittal sinus; ⑩ occipital lobe; ⑪ temporal lobe; ⑫ parietal lobe; ⑬ frontal lobe.

As seen from the lateral view on the insert, the scan shown in figures 20A and B passes through all four lobes—frontal, parietal, temporal, and occipital—which are separated by the central sulcus (C) and the sylvian fissure (S). The scan passes through the lowermost part of the parietal lobe and the uppermost part of the posterior temporal lobe.

The section extends through the body of the lateral ventricles. Anterior to the lateral ventricles, is the genu of the corpus callosum; the splenium lies posteriorly.

The falx is traversed by this section posteriorly. The length of the visualized falx indicates the approximate distance of this cut above the torcular.

Even at this high level, the uppermost part of the caudate nucleus is still visible just to the side of the lateral ventricle. Lateral to the caudate nucleus lies the corona radiata, formed by the fibers of the internal capsule.

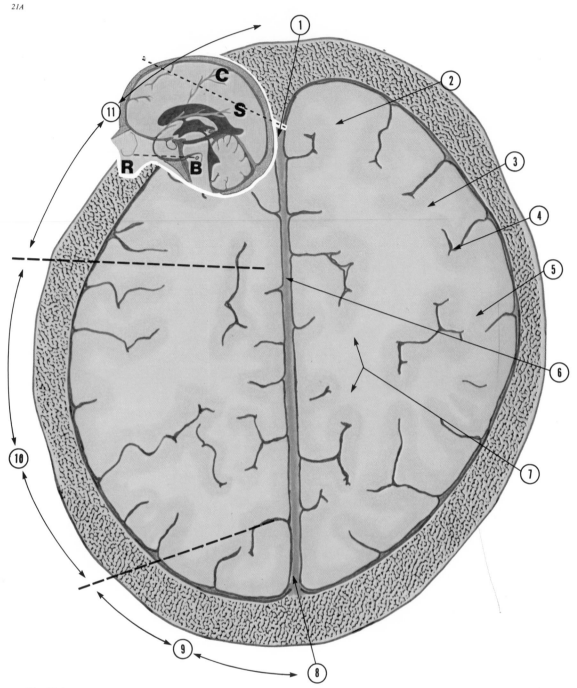

Fig. 21.A.
① superior sagittal sinus; ② superior frontal gyrus; ③ precentral gyrus; ④ central sulcus; ⑤ postcentral gyrus; ⑥ falx cerebri; ⑦ centrum semiovale; ⑧ superior sagittal sinus; ⑨ occipital lobe; ⑩ parietal lobe; ⑪ frontal lobe.

At the high level of the section shown in figures 21A and B, a landmark to separate the frontal, parietal, and occipital lobes is lacking. It is obvious, from the insert in figure 21A that a scan with a steep angulation covers only a small portion, while a scan with less angulation covers a greater portion of the frontal lobe.

For complete coverage of the brain, the highest scan must reach the cranial vault. Termination of the study at the level of that of figure 21B will miss a significant portion of the high convexity and parasagittal territory.

Recent technical advances in both hardware and software components, have resulted in the improved resolution of CT

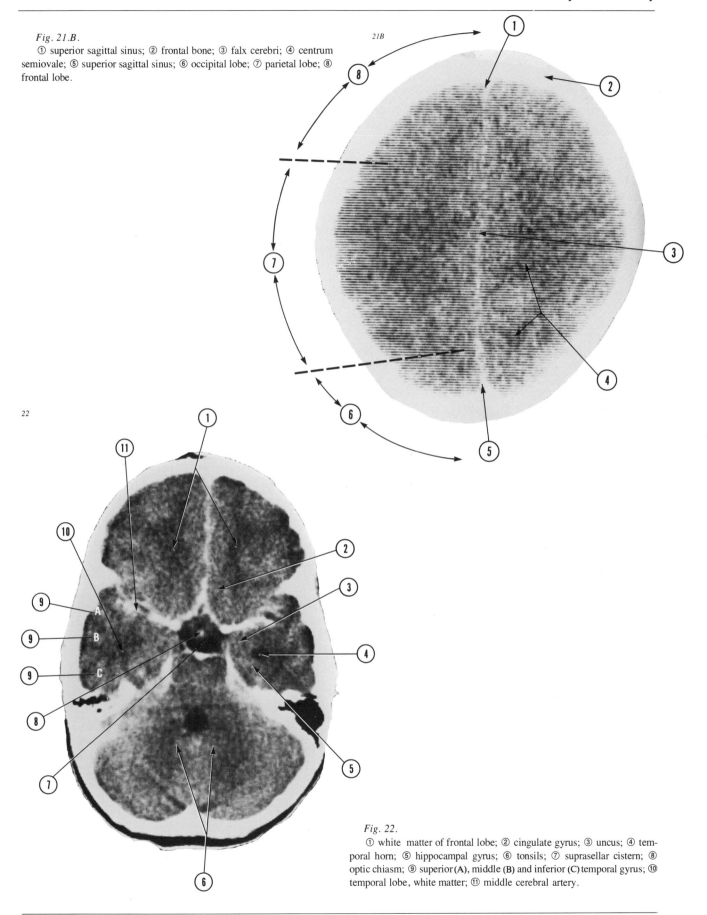

Fig. 21.B.
① superior sagittal sinus; ② frontal bone; ③ falx cerebri; ④ centrum semiovale; ⑤ superior sagittal sinus; ⑥ occipital lobe; ⑦ parietal lobe; ⑧ frontal lobe.

Fig. 22.
① white matter of frontal lobe; ② cingulate gyrus; ③ uncus; ④ temporal horn; ⑤ hippocampal gyrus; ⑥ tonsils; ⑦ suprasellar cistern; ⑧ optic chiasm; ⑨ superior (A), middle (B) and inferior (C) temporal gyrus; ⑩ temporal lobe, white matter; ⑪ middle cerebral artery.

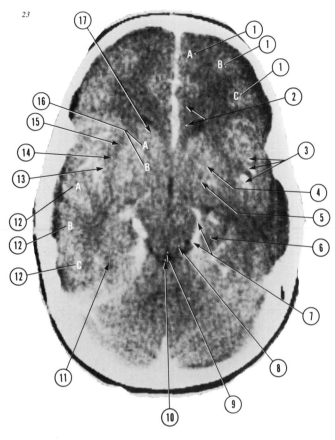

23

images. It is now possible to discriminate the gray matter, the white matter, the basal ganglia, the thalami, the internal and external capsules, and various gyri (figs. 22–27) (courtesy of LeRoy M. Kotzen, MD).

The anatomy of subarachnoid spaces can also be better delineated by intrathecal enhancement, using the water soluble nonionic contrast agent metrizamide (figs. 28 and 29). The contrast material can be injected either via the lumbar route or via direct C 1–2 puncture. If the lumbar route is chosen, the puncture is performed with a 22-gauge needle, with the patient in prone position. About 8 ml of metrizamide, at an iodide concentration of 170mg/ml, is instilled intrathecally. The table is tilted to a −60° Trendelenburg position, left there for 1–2 minutes, and then returned to a −10° position. The patient is then transferred on a similarly inclined stretcher for immediate CT scanning. Metrizamide enhanced computed tomography is especially suitable for studying small lesions in the sellar and juxtasellar region, the brainstem, and the posterior fossa territory.

Fig. 23.

① frontal gyrus—superior (A) middle (B) and inferior (C); ② cingulate gyrus; ③ middle cerebral arteries; ④ putamen; ⑤ globus pallidus; ⑥ hippocampal gyrus; ⑦ ambient cistern with enhanced posterior cerebral artery; ⑧ inferior colliculus; ⑨ aqueduct; ⑩ quadrigeminal cistern; ⑪ collateral sulcus; ⑫ temporal gyrus—(A) superior, (B) middle, and (C) inferior; ⑬ insula; ⑭ claustrum; ⑮ external capsule; ⑯ internal capsule—(A) anterior limb and (B) posterior limb; ⑰ caudate nucleus.

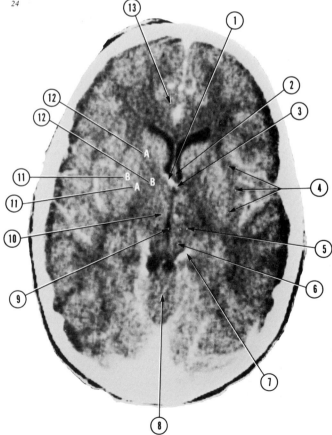

24

Fig. 24.

① thalamostriate vein; ② anterior column of fornix; ③ internal cerebral vein; ④ external capsule; ⑤ cerebral peduncle; ⑥ midbrain, tegmentum; ⑦ ambient cistern with enhanced vessels; ⑧ superior vermis; ⑨ third ventricle; ⑩ thalamus; ⑪ lenticular nucleus—(A) globus pallidus and (B) putamen; ⑫ internal capsule—(A) anterior limb and (B) posterior limb; ⑬ cingulate gyrus.

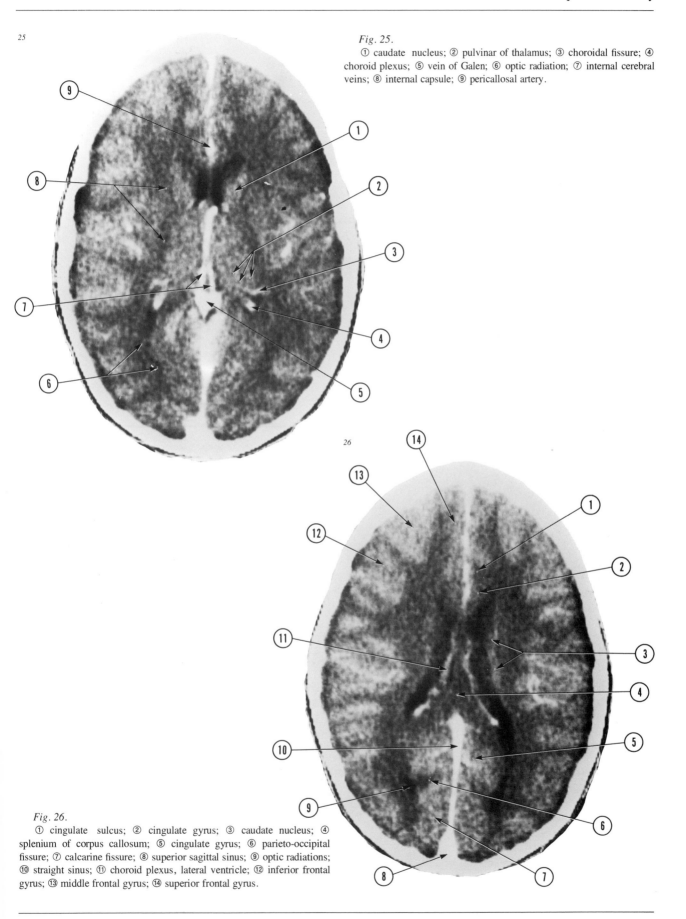

Fig. 25.

① caudate nucleus; ② pulvinar of thalamus; ③ choroidal fissure; ④ choroid plexus; ⑤ vein of Galen; ⑥ optic radiation; ⑦ internal cerebral veins; ⑧ internal capsule; ⑨ pericallosal artery.

Fig. 26.

① cingulate sulcus; ② cingulate gyrus; ③ caudate nucleus; ④ splenium of corpus callosum; ⑤ cingulate gyrus; ⑥ parieto-occipital fissure; ⑦ calcarine fissure; ⑧ superior sagittal sinus; ⑨ optic radiations; ⑩ straight sinus; ⑪ choroid plexus, lateral ventricle; ⑫ inferior frontal gyrus; ⑬ middle frontal gyrus; ⑭ superior frontal gyrus.

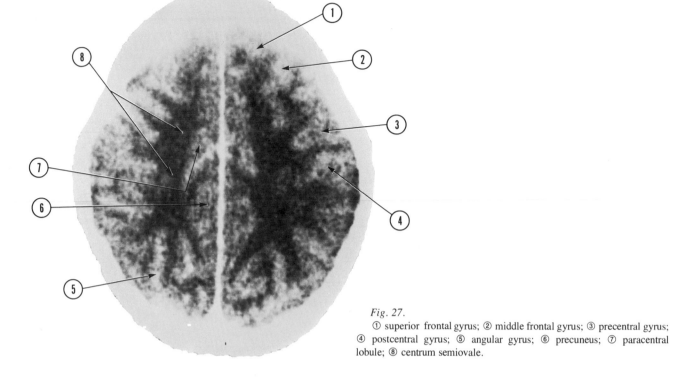

Fig. 27.

① superior frontal gyrus; ② middle frontal gyrus; ③ precentral gyrus; ④ postcentral gyrus; ⑤ angular gyrus; ⑥ precuneus; ⑦ paracentral lobule; ⑧ centrum semiovale.

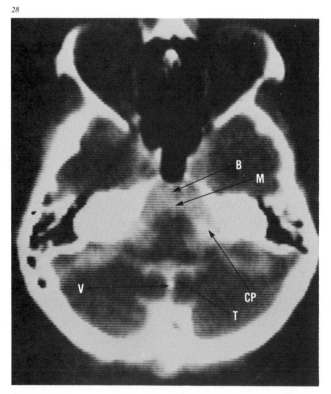

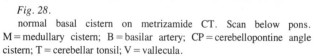

Fig. 28.

normal basal cistern on metrizamide CT. Scan below pons. M = medullary cistern; B = basilar artery; CP = cerebellopontine angle cistern; T = cerebellar tonsil; V = vallecula.

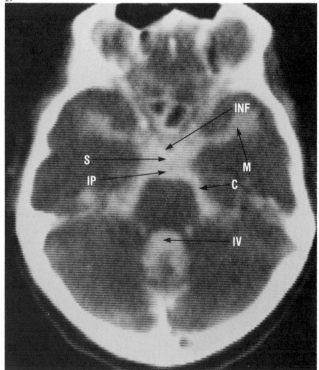

Fig. 29.

normal basal cistern on metrizamide CT. Scan through the pons. InF = infundibulum of pituitary; S = suprasellar cistern; IP = interpeduncular cistern; C = crural cistern; M = sylvian cistern (cistern of the middle cerebral artery); IV = fourth ventricle.

Bibliography

Carter BL, Morehead J, Wolpert SM, et al: Cross-sectional anatomy computed tomography and ultrasound correlation. Appleton-Century-Crofts, New York, 1977.

Di Chiro G: An Atlas of Detailed Normal Pneumoencephalographic Anatomy. CC Thomas, Springfield, 1961.

Drayer BP, Rosenbaum AE, Kennerdell JS, et al: Computed tomographic diagnosis of suprasellar masses by intrathecal enhancement. Radiology 123:339, 1977.

Drayer BP, Rosenbaum AE, Maroon JC, et al: Posterior fossa extraaxial cyst: diagnosis with metrizamide CT cisternography. AJR 128:431, 1977.

Gado M, Hanaway J, Frank R: Functional anatomy of the cerebral cortex by computed tomography. J Compt Assist Tomogr 3:1, 1979.

Glanz S, Geehr RB, Duncan CC, et al: Metrizamide-enhanced CT for evaluation of brainstem tumors. AJR 134:821, 1980.

Hayman LA, Evans RA, Hinck VC: Delayed high iodine dose contrast computed tomography. Radiology 136:677, 1980.

Liliequist B: The subarachnoid cisterns: an anatomic and roentgenologic study. Acta Radiol Suppl 185:1, 1959.

Manelfe, C, Clanet M, Giguad M: Internal capsule: normal anatomy and ischemic changes demonstrated by computed tomography. AJNR 2:149, 1981.

Naidich TP, Leeds NE, Kricheff II, et al: The tentorium in axial section I. Normal CT appearance and non-neoplastic pathology. Radiology 123:631, 1977.

New PFJ, Scott WR: Computed tomography of the brain and orbit (EMI scanning). Williams and Wilkins, Baltimore, 1975.

Norman D, Axel L, Berninger WH, et al: Dynamic computed tomography of the brain: techniques, data analysis, and applications. AJNR 2:1, 1981.

Peerkopf E: Atlas of Topographical and Applied Human Anatomy. Edited by Ferner H. WB Saunders, Philadelphia, 1963.

Roberts M, Hanaway J: Atlas of the Human Brain in Section. Lea and Febiger, Philadelphia, 1970.

Roberts PA, Claveria LE, Moseley IF: Computerized axial tomography and the normal brain. European seminar on computerized axial tomography in clinical practice. Edited by du Boulay GH, Moseley IF. Springer, Berlin, 1977.

Scott W, Hanaway J, Strother C: Atlas of the human brain and orbit for computed tomography. Warren H Green, St. Louis, 1976.

Takase M, Tolunga A, Otani K, et al: Atlas of the human brain for computed tomography based on the glabella-inion line. Neuroradiology 14:73, 1977.

Tokunga A, Takase M, Otani K: The glabella-inion line as a baseline for CT scanning of the brain. Neuroradiology 14:67, 1977.

Wing SD, Anderson RE, Osborn AG: Dynamic cranial computed tomography: preliminary results. AJR 134:941, 1980.

Chapter III

Computed tomography is a reliable diagnostic method for detecting the affect of acute and chronic head injury. A fresh intracranial hematoma can be easily demonstrated, whether it lies in the epidural or subdural space or within the cerebral parenchyma, the ventricles, or cisterns. In general CT is superior to angiography not only because it localizes and shows the extent of the hematoma, but also because it is highly specific, capable of differentiating between hematoma and edema.

Acute Epidural and Subdural Hematomas

Fresh hematoma has an attenuation coefficient ranging from 40 to 100 HU (scale, 1000), which is considerably denser than that of the brain (white matter 29–31 HU; grey matter 30–35 HU) and cerebrospinal fluid (4 to 14 HU).

The increased density of extravasated blood (40 to 100 HU), compared to circulating blood (25 to 56 HU), is related to the protein component of tightly packed hemoglobin molecules. Iron and calcium contribute only minimally to the absorption values seen in a fresh blood clot.

Acute epidural hematoma is characterized as a biconvex, lentiform, homogeneous area of high density, well-demarcated from the underlying brain (fig. 30). CT is especially valuable and expedient in detecting a posterior fossa epidural hematoma, which may be quite difficult and time-consuming to diagnose angiographically (fig. 31 A and B).

Acute subdural hematoma is crescentic in shape (fig. 32). Its homogeneously high density is convex along the inner table, but concave against the brain. While epidural hematoma is limited by the dura, subdural hematoma spreads along a large potential subdural space and is usually slightly less dense than the epidural hematoma.

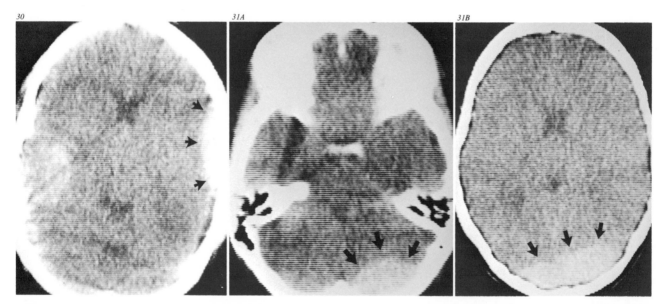

Fig. 30. Acute left temporal epidural hematoma. Note the characteristic biconvex high density fresh blood clot (*arrows*), homogeneous and dense, confluent with the inner table. No angiographic confirmation was necessary and the hematoma was evacuated surgically. Intracerebral hematoma with some edema in the right temporal lobe (angiographically confirmed). The area of high attenuation is not confluent with the inner table. It is less dense and less homogeneous than the left epidural hematoma. Notice the absence of ventricular shift due to bilateral lesions.

Fig. 31. Acute posterior fossa epidural hematoma. This 19-year-old student was hit by a car and fell backward, striking her occiput. She was

admitted for overnight observation. Skull radiographs showed no fracture and she was neurologically intact. But next morning, she suddenly deteriorated and had a respiratory arrest. She was resuscitated and an emergency CT revealed a posterior fossa epidural hematoma, which was immediately evacuated without additional study. The patient made an uneventful recovery.

A An epidural hematoma in the posterior fossa (*arrows*) is well shown.

B On higher section, the epidural hematoma extends above the tentorium and to the right side.

32

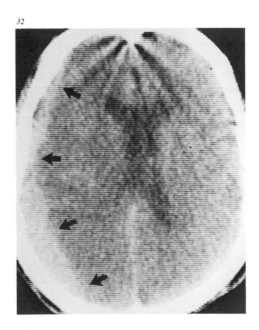

Fig. 32. Acute subdural hematoma. Note the high density zone with a convex outer margin along the inner table and a concave inner margin (*arrows*) along the underlying brain. It extends over a large area and exerts a diffuse pressure effect on the lateral ventricle.

33A

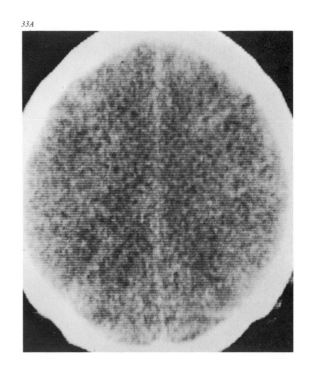

Isodense Subdural Hematoma

The high density of acute subdural hematoma persists for 2 to 3 weeks. Gradually, hemoglobin breaks down and cerebrospinal fluid enters the subdural space by osmosis. This process naturally decreases the attenuation value of the subacute subdural hematoma (2 to 3 weeks to 2 months old), which may appear isodense on CT, i.e., its density is the same as that of the underlying brain. If the subdural hematoma is isodense to the brain, CT may not detect it (fig. 33A). Contrast administration is strongly indicated, since it may enhance the membrane of the hematoma, which would make the diagnosis possible even though the hematoma itself is isodense (fig. 33B).

The upper scans should be scrutinized carefully for a displaced cortical vein, a subtle but important finding in diagnosing isodense subdural hematoma (fig. 34A–C).

Scans delayed 4 to 6 hours after contrast injection may enhance the isodense subdural hematoma.

A unilateral isodense or chronic subdural hematoma that causes significant midline shift may present some of the following characteristic ventricular deformities, which should arouse suspicion of subdural hematoma: (a) posterior displacement of the ipsilateral anterior horn; (b) compression of the ipsilateral posterior and temporal horns; (c) anterior displacement of the ipsilateral glomus of the choroid plexus; and (d) widening of the contralateral ventricle (fig. 35). Indeed, extracerebral hematoma must always be suspected

33B

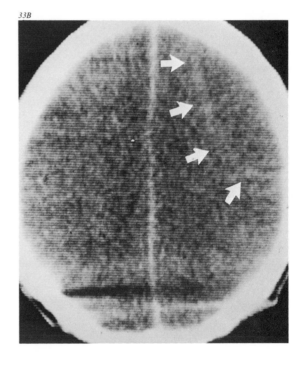

Fig. 33. Isodense chronic subdural hematoma, not visible on non-contrast scan.

A Noncontrast scan fails to distinguish the isodense subdural hematoma from the underlying brain tissue.

B Contrast scan. The membrane of the chronic subdural hematoma is outlined (*arrows*).

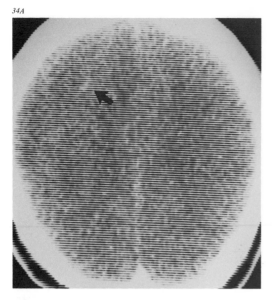

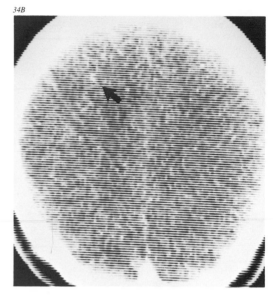

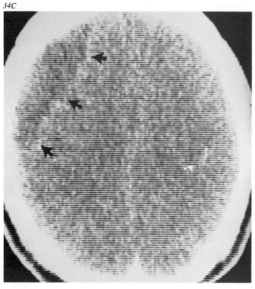

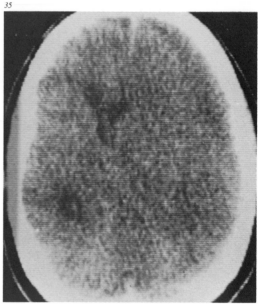

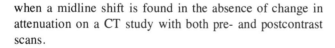

when a midline shift is found in the absence of change in attenuation on a CT study with both pre- and postcontrast scans.

Fig. 34. Isodense subdural hematoma visualized on contrast scans by displaced cortical vein as enhanced dot.

A and B Enhanced, displaced cortical vein (*arrows*) on two consecutive scans.

Chronic Subdural Hematoma

At the end of 2 to 3 months, the subdural hematoma becomes uniformly lucent and gives a typical low density CT appearance against the underlying brain (fig. 36). The shape of chronic subdural hematoma may vary from crescentic to biconvex. A rebleed may occur within a chronic subdural hematoma, and result in an admixture of high and low densities (fig. 37A and B). Occasionally, an interesting gravitational phenomenon is observed wherein the dense

C Repeat contrast scan 1-month later. Chronic subdural hematoma clearly seen with enhanced membrane (*arrows*).

Fig. 35. Large chronic subdural hematoma on the left, producing characteristic deformity of the ventricular system.

Fig. 36. Bilateral chronic subdural hematoma with posterior displacement of both frontal horns.

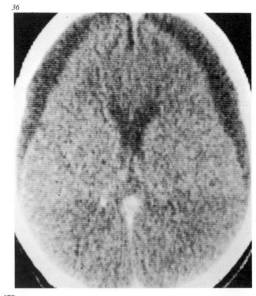

Fig. 37. A Chronic low density subdural hematoma with admixture of high density hematoma (*arrows*) probably due to recent rebleed. The blood settles into the dependent part of the subdural space. Bony defect on the left is due to craniotomy for berry aneurysm 13 years ago.

B Repeat scan 1 month later. Typical low density subdural hematoma. The lateral ventricles are now more dilated apparently due to the development of communicating hydrocephalus.

Fig. 38. Contusion edema. Scan 2 weeks after trauma showing contusion edema (*arrows*) in the right posterior temporal lobe.

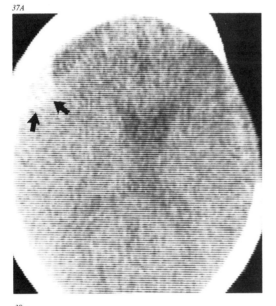

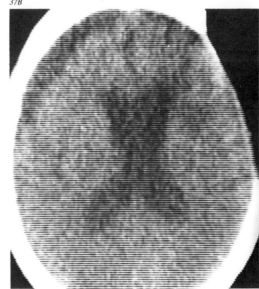

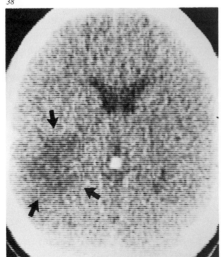

cells and debris layer-out in the lower part, while the lucent liquefied subdural hematoma remains on top.

Contusion Edema and Its Differential Diagnosis

CT demonstrates the effect of local contusion as a localized low density area that, unlike infarct, does not follow vascular distribution (fig. 38). A low-density, low-grade astrocytoma may also mimic contusion edema (see fig. 75). Serial studies, with and without contrast injection, may help to differentiate these two conditions.

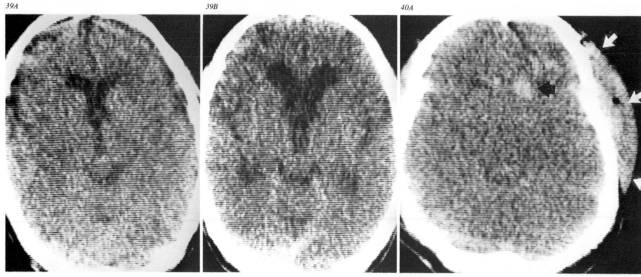

39A   *39B*   *40A*

Fig. 39. Development of communicating hydrocephalus after head trauma. A 63-year-old male was admitted with obtundation and multiple lacerations and broken ribs.

A   Admission scan reveals normal size ventricles. Lumbar puncture yielded grossly bloody fluid.

B   Repeat scan 1-month later reveals communicating hydrocephalus. Clinically the patient developed Korsakoff's psychosis.

Fig. 40. Depressed fractures not obvious on conventional window setting, but easily appreciated on wide window width.

A   Left frontal intracerebral hematoma (*black arrows*) and marked soft tissue swelling of the scalp (*white arrows*).

B   Same image as in *A*, but with wide window width showing depressed fractures (*white arrows*).

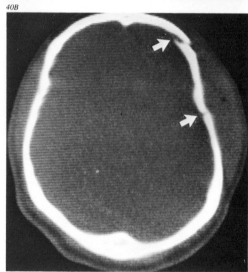

40B

Post-traumatic Communicating Hydrocephalus

The high sensitivity of CT permits the study of ventricular size and the cortical sulci. Because CT is noninvasive, it is especially suitable for serial studies to detect the early development of post-traumatic hydrocephalus (fig. 39A and B) and to assess the effectiveness of shunting procedures for communicating hydrocephalus.

Depressed Skull Fracture

While conventional radiography remains the choice of study for fracture of the skull, CT is ideal for evaluating the degree of the depressed fracture in relation to the normal calvarium. To evaluate the bony architecture, a wide window width, greater than 1000 HU, must be used (fig. 40 A and B).

Acute Isodense Subdural Hematoma

An acute subdural hematoma in an anemic patient with a hemoglobin value of 8–10 g/dl may be isodense on CT. This is because the density of hematoma is directly related to its hemoglobin concentration. Acute isodense subdural hematoma in anemic patients has been reported in both supratentorial and infratentorial regions.

Other supportive CT findings of isodense subdural hematoma are obliteration of the ipsilateral sulci, a midline shift, and ipsilateral ventricular compression. At times, arteriography may be the only way to resolve the problem (fig. 41A–C).

Delayed Traumatic Intracranial Hematoma

In patients suffering from severe head injury, delayed intracranial hematoma, not observed on initial CT, may de-

41A

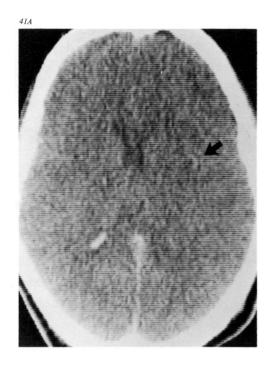

41B

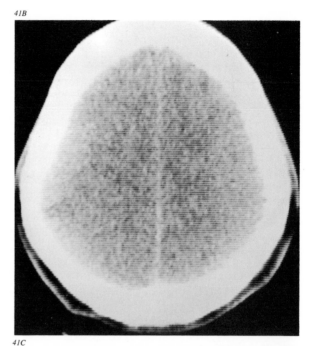

41C

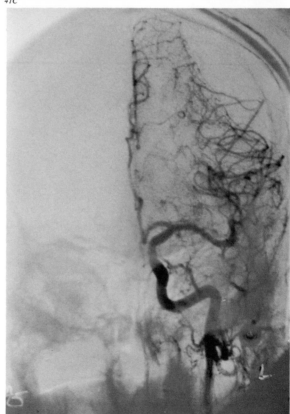

Fig. 41. Bilateral isodense subdural hematoma. This 84-year-old man, had a 3-week history of persistent headache following a head injury. When admitted to the hospital, there was no focal neurologic finding. Post-contrast scans showed:

A A slight midline shift to the right side. Both lateral ventricles were abnormally small for a patient of this age. A small dot-like density (*arrow*) raises the question of a medially displaced cortical vein, but this impression is not definite.

B Scan at a higher level reveals obliteration of sulci on both sides. Although the diagnosis of bilateral subdural hematoma was suspected on CT study, an angiogram was performed for confirmation.

C Left carotid arteriogram reveals a large chronic subdural hematoma with only slight shift of the anterior cerebral artery. Surgery confirmed bilateral chronic subdural hematoma.

velop. Delayed intracerebral hematoma may be due to local failure of mechanisms that regulate cerebral blood flow following a severe contusional injury. This failure of cerebral blood flow regulation may result in diapedesis and hematoma formation. Most delayed intracerebral hematomas are detected within 48 hours following head injury and are associated with a poor outcome.

Delayed unilateral extra-axial collections may occur contralateral to the site of injury and follow surgical decompression. It thus appears that surgical relief of tamponade may play a role in causing these collections. Delayed extra-axial collections may also be due to effusion from diffuse brain injection and arachnoidal tears.

Bibliography

Ambrose J: Computerized transverse axial scanning (tomography): Part II. Clinical application. Br J Radiol 46:1023, 1973.

Ambrose J, Gooding MR, Uttley D: EMI scans in the management of head injuries. Lancet 1:847, 1976.

Amendola MA, Ostrum BJ: Diagnosis of isodense subdural hematomas by computed tomography. AJR 129:693, 1977.

Davis KR, Taveras JM, Roberson GH, et al: Computed tomography in head trauma. Semin Roentgenol 12:53, 1977.

Dublin AB, French BN, Rennick JM: Computed tomography in head trauma. Radiology 122:365, 1977.

Forbes GS, Sheedy PF, Plepgras DG, et al: Computed tomography in the evaluation of subdural hematomas. Radiology 126:143, 1978.

Kim KS, Hemmati J, Weinberg PE: Computed tomography in isodense subdural hematoma. Radiology 128:71, 1978.

Koo AH: Evaluation of head trauma by computed tomography. Radiology 123:345, 1977.

Lavender B, Stattin S, Svendsen P: Computer tomography of traumatic intra- and extracerebral lesions. Acta Radiol Suppl 346:107, 1975.

Lipper MH, Kishore PRS, Girevendulis AK, et al: Delayed intracranial hematoma in patients with severe head injury. Radiology 133:645, 1979.

Möller A, Ericson K: Computed tomography of isoattenuating subdural hematomas. Radiology 130:149, 1979.

Merino-de-Villasante J, Taveras J: Computerized tomography (CT) in acute head trauma. AJR 126:765, 1976.

Messina AV: Computed tomography: contrast media within subdural hematomas. A preliminary report. Radiology 119:725, 1976.

Messina AV, Chernik NL: Computed tomography: the "resolving" intracerebral hemorrhage. Radiology 118:609, 1975.

Naidich TP: Trauma. Computed tomography. Edited by Norman D, Korobkin M, Newton T. Springer, Berlin, 1977.

New PFJ, Scott WR: Computed tomography of the brain and orbit (EMI scanning). Williams and Wilkins, Baltimore, 1975.

Paxton R, Ambrose J: The EMI scanning: a brief review of the first 650 patients. Br J Radiol 47:530, 1974.

Rieth KG, Schwartz FT, Davis DO: Acute isodense epidural hematoma on computed tomography. J Comput Assist Tomogr 3:691, 1979.

Scotti G, Terrugge K, Melancon D, et al: Evaluation of the age of subdural hematomas by computerized tomography. J Neurosurg 47:311, 1977.

Smith WP, Batnitzky SB, Rengachary SS: Acute isodense subdural hematomas: a problem in anemic patients. AJR 136:543, 1981.

Snoeck J, Jennett B, Adams JH, et al: Computerized tomography after recent severe head injury in patients without acute intracranial hematoma. J Neurol Neurosurg Psychiatry 42:215, 1979.

Tsai FY, Huprich JE, Gardner FC, et al: Diagnostic and prognostic implications of computed tomography of head trauma. J Comput Assist Tomogr 2:323, 1978.

Tsai FY, Teal JS, Quinn MF, et al: CT of brainstem injury. AJR 134:717, 1980.

Chapter IV

Computed tomography is a safe and preferred method for diagnosing cerebral infarction. When the differentiation between cerebral infarction and hemorrhage is difficult but important clinically for the management of patients with possible anticoagulant therapy, CT distinguishes between them without difficulty.

It is important, however, to realize the limitation of CT in cerebral infarction, since at least one-third of infarctions may escape detection if only a single study is performed. It has been reported that CT within 24 hours of admission detects only 58 percent of patients with infarction, and only two-thirds of patients with infarct reveal positive CT findings in 7 to 10 days. In another series it was found that within the first 12 hours of cerebral infarction, the CT is usually normal. From then on, and up to 48 hours after the infarction, about one-half of the patients have an abnormal

Computed Tomography in Cerebral Infarction

CT. Repeat examination after 2 to 4 days increases the positive CT to about 75 percent.

The CT changes in cerebral infarction vary from the acute swelling stage to the stage of healing (figs. 42–47).

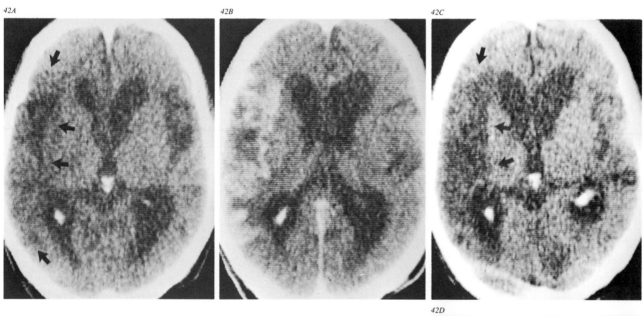

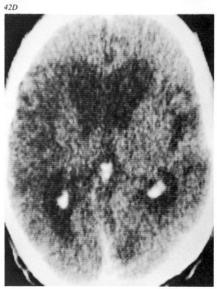

Fig. 42. Change of contrast enhancement with age of infarct. Right middle cerebral infarct in a 71-year-old man who presented with left hemiplegia. Scans on day 5:

A Precontrast scan reveals the low density area in the distribution of the right middle cerebral artery is only poorly demarcated from its surrounding tissue (*arrows*).

B Postcontrast scan. Margin-like zones of increased attenuation are visible around the infarcted area. Some pressure effect on the right frontal horn is discernible.

C and D Scans on day 17. Precontrast scan (*C*) shows low density infarct sharply demarcated from neighboring brain (*arrows*).

D Postcontrast scan shows infarcted area is slightly enhanced so that its distinction from the normal becomes less obvious.

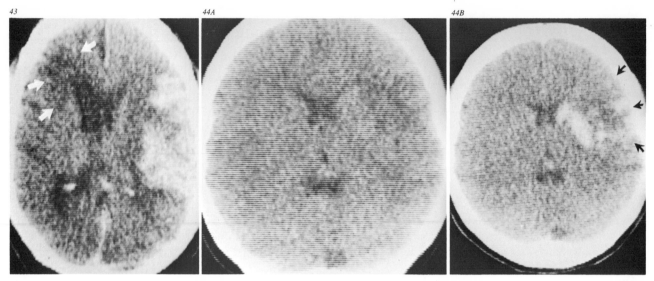

Fig. 43. Contrast scan on day 7. Note enhanced left middle cerebral infarction. There is also an old infarct in the right frontal lobe (*arrows*).

Fig. 44. Enhanced left middle cerebral artery infarction, involving the cortical area and the basal ganglia. This 44-year-old hypertensive female presented with sudden onset of right hemiparesis. Scans on day 9—

A Precontrast scan reveals the only abnormality is a low density area lateral to the caudate nucleus, which appears normal in comparison with the opposite side.

B Postcontrast scan reveals enhancement actually involves both the caudate and lentiform nucleus as well as the cortex (*arrows*). Without contrast injection, involvement of the caudate and lentiform nucleus would not be detectable. This case clearly demonstrates the value of contrast injection in the study of infarction.

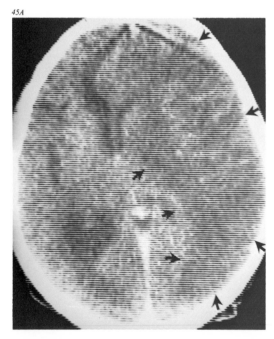
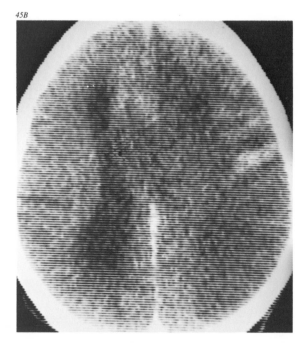

Fig. 45. Massive left carotid infarction. An 81-year-old hypertensive and diabetic female was admitted with sudden onset of right hemiparesis and left focal seizures that progressed rapidly to obtundation. Contrast scan on day 8 shows left carotid artery occlusion with massive infarct.

A The entire vascular supply of the left anterior and middle cerebral artery is visualized by a homogeneous area of decreased density (*arrows*). Note extension of low density into both grey and white matter. Only the supply of the posterior cerebral artery is spared. Mass effect with ventricular encroachment and midline shift is striking.

B Diffuse extension of edema into the white and grey matter is to be distinguished from perifocal edema involving the white matter and is seen in brain tumors. Some finger-like enhancement is noted. Patient died 2 months after scan.

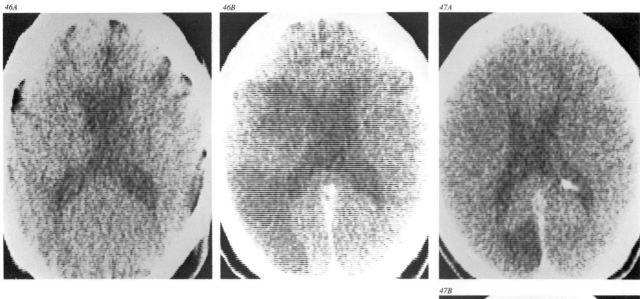

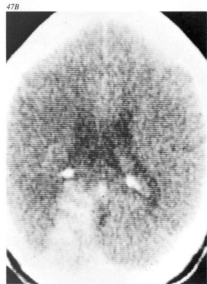

Fig. 46. Value of repeat scan even with only 3-day interval in a 72-year-old male who developed a sudden change in mental status with impaired memory and dysphasia.

A Scan on day 5 shows slight motion but no obvious lesion.

B Repeat scan 3 days later reveals typical fan-shaped middle cerebral artery infarct is now well demarcated from the normal posterior cerebral territory. Anteriorly the infarct extends to the parietal lobe, compressing on the lateral ventricle.

Fig. 47. Classic appearance of a fresh and an old posterior cerebral infarct.

A Contrast scan shows enhanced infarct in the territory of the right posterior cerebral artery with mass effect displacing the choroid plexus forward.

B Contrast scan of the same infarct, now 2½ months old, shows well-delineated nonenhanced, low density lesion due to old infarct in posterior cerebral artery territory.

Acute Swelling Stage

This state may last from a few days to a few weeks. The infarct appears either normal or as an area of slightly decreased attenuation, which is only poorly delineated and marginated from surrounding tissues. The low density is probably due to tissue swelling and corresponds with vascular territory. Seventy percent of the lesion occurs in the distribution of the middle cerebral artery.

Resorption Stage

The second stage may last for weeks or months. Usually, by the end of the first week, the edema regresses. In this stage, the process of tissue breakdown and phagocytosis, and the removal of dead tissue by macrophages continues. The area becomes better demarcated from surrounding tissue.

The infarct in the first stage has more of the affect of a space-occupying mass than in the resorption stage, where some shrinking of the hypodense area is beginning to be seen.

Healing Stage

The infarct may go on healing, and through regeneration and revascularization, normal tissue parenchyma may replace the infarcted area and the CT returns completely to normal. On the other hand, liquefaction and necrosis may take place so that small defects or encephalomalacic cystic cavities, containing fluid with the same density as cerebro-

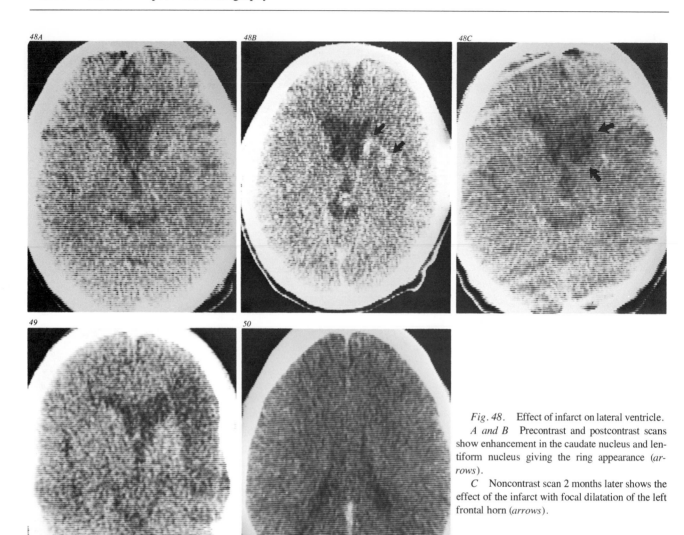

48A   *48B*   *48C*

Fig. 48. Effect of infarct on lateral ventricle.

A and B Precontrast and postcontrast scans show enhancement in the caudate nucleus and lentiform nucleus giving the ring appearance (*arrows*).

C Noncontrast scan 2 months later shows the effect of the infarct with focal dilatation of the left frontal horn (*arrows*).

Fig. 49. A typical case of old left middle cerebral artery infarct. Note the well-defined low attenuation lesion in the left frontotemporal region, a territory of the middle cerebral artery, the dilatation of the left frontal horn, and the ipsilateral shift of both lateral ventricles and the third ventricle.

Fig. 50. Ring-enhanced infarct with triangular, perifocal edema. Differentiation from metastasis, malignant glioma, and abscess may be difficult on single examination.

spinal fluid, may develop. By 4 to 8 weeks, if the area of liquefaction necrosis is of sufficient size, the adjacent ventricular part may deviate toward the defect, resulting in a midline shift toward the infarct with ipsilateral ventricular dilatation (figs. 48 and 49).

Injection of Iodinated Contrast Medium

The pattern and degree of enhancement varies greatly from very faint to highly dense and from band-like and finger-like to ring-like enhancement (fig. 50). The latter must be differentiated from malignant glioma, metastasis, and abscess (see figs. 77B, 87B, and 89B). In cases of doubt, serial study and angiography may be employed.

A mass effect in recent infarction is common, and the presence of mass effect with enhancement may be misdiagnosed as neoplasm or abscess (fig. 51). One important criterion for infarct is the regression of the edema and mass effect within 2 to 3 weeks after the onset of symptoms. Persistence of edema around an enhanced lesion should arouse suspicion of either neoplasm or abscess.

It is generally agreed that CT will demonstrate infarction in the first week in more patients than does radionuclide scanning. The radionuclide scan, however, may reveal some infarctions not demonstrated by the CT.

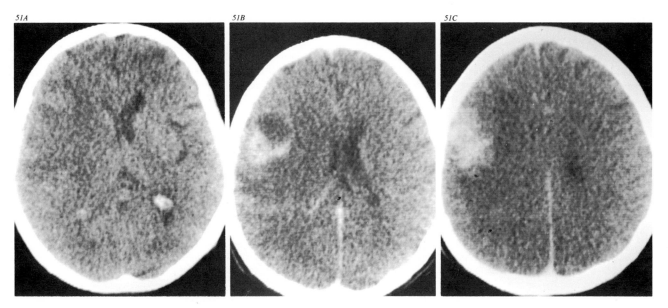

Fig. 51. An example of ring-enhanced infarct with mass effect misdiagnosed as neoplasm in a 73-year-old man. He had been admitted with onset of periphery 7th nerve paresis on the left, decrease of taste sensation 5 weeks ago, sudden onset of left hemiparesis with sensory deficit, and gait disturbances. Chest radiograph was reported to reveal a "mass" lesion.

A Precontrast scan shows low attenuation mass in the right frontotemporal area with marked compression of the right frontal horn and

contralateral shift of the ventricular system. The right choroid plexus is displaced posteriorly.

B and C Postcontrast scans at slightly higher levels show marked enhancement with nodularity and ring associated with edema and mass effect. Clinically the lesion was thought to represent metastasis, which was found to be an infarct at surgery.

Fig. 52. An example of right cerebellar infarct in a 56-year-old woman who was brought to the emergency room with a history of vertigo, headache, and unsteady gait for 4 days. Examination revealed incoordination of the right arm and a positive Romberg sign.

A and B Pre- and postcontrast scans revealed a nonenhanced low density lesion in the high right cerebellar hemisphere extending to the vermis (*arrows*). This was consistent with an infarction of the territory of the superior cerebellar artery. No hydrocephalus was noted on higher scans.

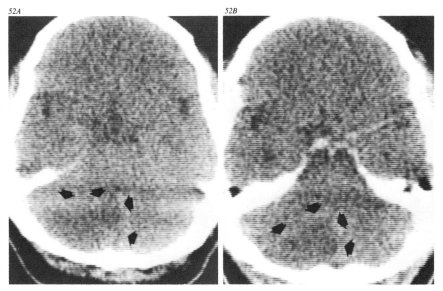

Infarction of the Brainstem and Cerebellum

While CT is useful in diagnosing infarctions in the posterior fossa, it is not as sensitive as scans in the supratentorial region (fig. 52). Even with scanners of the latest model, artifacts at the skull base are numerous and a small infarct may be missed. Further technical improvement in the territory of the posterior fossa is necessary.

Bibliography

Aulich A, Wende S, Fenski A, et al: Diagnosis and follow-up studies in cerebral infarcts. In: Cranial Computerized Tomography. Edited by Lanksch W, Kazner E. Springer, Berlin, 1976.

Campbell JK, Houser OW, Stevens JC, et al: Computed tomography and radionuclide imaging in the evaluation of ischemic stroke. Radiology 126:695, 1978.

Constant P, Renou AM, Caille JM, et al: CAT studies of cerebral ischemia. European seminar on computerized axial tomography in clinical practice. Edited by de Boulay GH, Moseley IF. Springer, Berlin, 1977.

Cronqvist S, Brismar J, Kjellin K, et al: Computer assisted axial tomography in cerebrovascular lesions. Acta Radiol 16:135, 1975.

Davis KR, Taveras JM, New PFM, et al: Cerebral infarction diagnosis by computerized tomography. AJR 124:643, 1975.

Drayer BP, Dujovny M, Boehnke M, et al: The capacity for computed tomography diagnosis of cerebral infarction: an experimental study in the nonhuman primate. Radiology 125:393, 1977.

Harrison MJG: The use of CAT in cerebral infarction. European seminar on computerized axial tomography in clinical practice. Edited by du Boulay GH, Moseley IF. Springer, Berlin, 1977, pp 221–226.

Hinshaw DB, Thompson JR, Hasso AN, et al: Infarctions of the brainstem and cerebellum: a correlation of computed tomography and angiography. Radiology 137:105, 1980.

Inoue Y, Takemoto K. Miyamoto T, et al:Sequential computed tomography scans in acute cerebral infarction. Radiology 135:655, 1980.

Kendall BE, Pullicino P: Intravascular contrast injection in ischaemic lesions. II. Effect on prognosis. Neuroradiology 19:241, 1980.

Lassen NA: The luxury perfusion syndrome. Lancet 2:1113, 1966.

Lee KF, Chambers RA, Park DC, et al: Evaluation of cerebral infarction by CT with special emphasis on microinfarction. Neuroradiology 16:156, 1978.

Lukin RR, Chamber AA, Tomsich TA: Cerebral vascular lesions: infarction, hemorrhage, aneurysm, and arteriovenous malformation. Semin Roentgenol 12:77, 1977.

New PFJ, Scott WR: Computed tomography of the brain and orbit (EMI scanning). Williams and Wilkins, Baltimore, 1975.

Palmers Y, Staelens B, Baert AL et al: Cerebral ischemia. In: Clinical Computer Tomography—Head and Trunk. Edited by Baert A, Jeanmart L, Wackenheim A. Springer, Berlin, pp 113–127.

Paxton R, Ambrose J: The EMI scanner: a brief review of the first 650 patients. Br J Radiol 47:530, 1974.

Pollock JA: Stroke. In: Computed Tomography. Edited by Norman D, Korobkin M, Newton TH. CV Mosby, 1977, pp 255–262.

Pullicino P, Kendall BE: Contrast enhancement in ischaemic lesions. I. Relationship to prognosis. Neuroradiology 19:235, 1980.

Weisberg LA: Computerized tomographic enhancement pattern in cerebral infarction. Arch Neurol 37:21, 1980.

Wing SD, Norman D, Pollock JA, et al: Contrast enhancement of cerebral infarcts in computed tomography. Radiology 121:89, 1976.

Yock DH, Marshall WH Jr: Recent ischemic brain infarcts at computed tomography. Appearances pre- and postcontrast infusion. Radiology 117:599, 1975.

Yock D, Norman D, Newton TH: Pitfalls in the diagnosis of ischemic cerebral infarcts by computed tomography. In: The diagnostic Limitations of Computerized Axial Tomography. Edited by Bories J. Springer, Berlin, 1978, pp 90–104.

Chapter V

Intracerebral Hemorrhage

Before the era of computerized tomography, intracerebral hematoma could not be diagnosed with certainty. Conventional neuroradiologic methods, such as angiography and air study, would only reveal the mass effect of the hematoma, which could not be differentiated from that of cerebral infarction or any avascular mass. Computerized tomography permits sensitive soft tissue distinction and thus, for the first time, makes a specific diagnosis of intracerebral hematoma possible.

The density of the fresh intracerebral hematoma measures 40 to 100 HU (20 to 50 EMI units). Approximately 60 percent of intracerebral hematomas are due to trauma or hypertension, 25 percent to ruptured aneurysms or arteriovenous malformations, and 15 percent to miscellaneous causes, including anticoagulation therapy.

CT demonstrates acute blood within the brain parenchyma, the ventricles, and the basal cisterns (figs. 53 and 54). In acute intracerebral hematoma, only a thin layer of perihematoma lucency is seen, due to extravasation of serum from the blood clot or perifocal edema.

Based on the extent and distribution of the hemorrhage, prognosis can be accurately predicted. But a limited extent of the hematoma does not necessarily preclude a grave outcome, since its location also plays a vital role in this respect (fig. 55).

In the pre-CT era, mortality from intracerebral hemorrhage was estimated to be as high as 75–95 percent. The mortality from intracerebral hemorrhage based on CT is, however, only 30 percent.

The precise location of the hematoma influences the decision for surgical evacuation (fig. 56), a process made easier by CT, which provides information heretofore unobtainable.

While the acute hematoma presents no diagnostic problem on CT, hematoma evolving between 2 weeks and 2 or 3 months may present a problem in differential diagnosis with neoplasm, abscess, or infarct (figs. 57–63). This problem is increased if no initial CT is performed for comparison immediately following hemorrhage, or if the patient's history is inadequate.

During the stage of resolution, two possibilities may lead to the erroneous diagnosis of a resolving hematoma as some other condition: (a) the high absorption value in acute hematoma remains high for at least 2 weeks. Gradually, elements within the clot become necrotic and breakdown products are being absorbed. At one stage, the "resolved" blood becomes isodense. CT at this time will reveal the effect of edema on the ventricles—i.e., a midline shift and ventricular displacement without the typical appearance of the high density blood clot. The glioma would be very difficult to differentiate from this stage of "resolving" hematoma. (b) Between 2 weeks and 2 to 3 months after intra-

Computed Tomography in Intracerebral Hemorrhage, Arteriovenous Malformation, and Aneurysm

cerebral hemorrhage, new capillaries are formed in the perihematoma edematous region. These newly formed vessels have an abormal blood-brain barrier and cause extra-

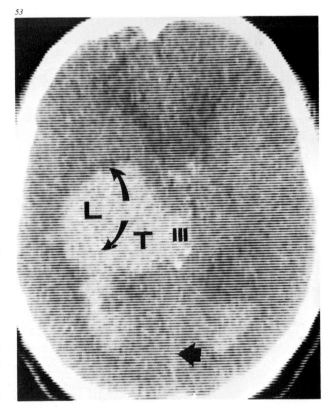

Fig. 53. Hypertensive thalamic and lentiform hemorrhage in a 70-year-old hypertensive man who developed progressive loss of consciousness. He had become rapidly stuporous with left hemiplegia, and comatose with brainstem reflexes only. A noncontrast scan on the day of ictus showed a high density hemorrhage in the thalamus (T), internal capsule (*arrows*), lentiform nucleus (L), third ventricle (III), both occipital horns, and the interhemispheric fissure (*arrow*). Due to the acuteness of the lesion, there is only minimal edema anterior to the ganglionic hematoma. The patient died the next day.

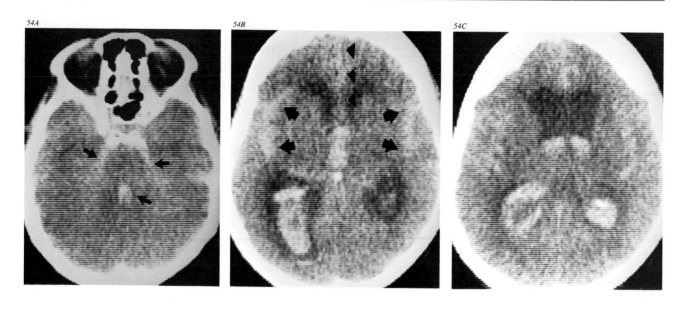

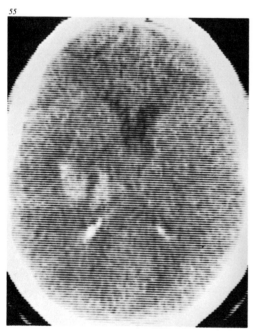

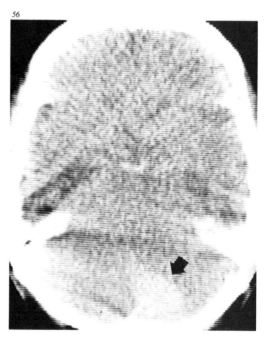

Fig. 54. Hypertensive subarachnoid hemorrhage in a 69-year-old woman who had fallen and struck her head. In the emergency room, she was able to give her history, but rapidly became unresponsive. She died the next day. Noncontrast CT was performed on the day of ictus. Three selected scans reveal:

A High density, fresh hematoma within the fourth ventricle and perimesencephalic cisterns (*arrows*);

B Fresh hematoma in the interhemispheric fissure (*arrowheads*), both sylvian fissures (*arrows*), the third ventricle, and the right occipital horn;

C Hematoma in both frontal and occipital horns.

Fig. 55. Hypertensive ganglionic hematoma. Acute hematoma in the posterior lateral thalamus and posterior putamen of a hypertensive 65-year-old woman who had been injured in a fight. When brought to the emergency room, she was sitting in a chair and yelling. This behavior

progressed to progressively increasing lethargy and unresponsiveness. Noncontrast scan on day 3 revealed an acute hematoma in the posterior thalamus, extending laterally to involve the posterior putamen. There is pressure effect on the right frontal horn with only minimal shift. The patient died 6 days after CT.

Fig. 56. Hypertensive hematoma in the left cerebellar hemisphere (surgically removed) of a 37-year-old man with chronic hypertension who developed seizures, headache, and vomiting, which began suddenly. The family said he lost his balance on standing up. In the emergency room he was lethargic and disoriented, without focal neurologic findings. Lumbar puncture was grossly bloody. His blood pressure was 225/140 mmHg. A noncontrast scan on day 2 showed triangular high density fresh hematoma in the left cerebellar hemisphere. Higher cuts demonstrate moderate triventricular dilatation. On admission, there was skew deviation of his eyes. He was increasingly obtunded, and at surgery 20 ml of blood was evacuated. This patient made an uneventful recovery.

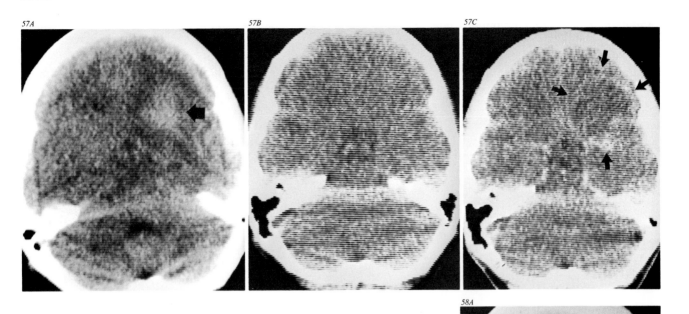

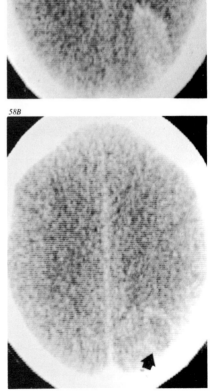

Fig. 57. Resolving hematoma mistaken as high density tumor on outside scan in a 32-year old woman who developed sudden left frontal headache with nausea and vomiting. A lumbar puncture was clear.

A Outside noncontrast CT on day 23 reveals a high density lesion surrounded by edema with mass effect (*arrow*) and ventricular shift on higher cuts (not shown). This high density lesion was thought to represent a neoplasm. A radionuclide scan was class IV positive in the left frontal lobe region. The patient was referred for a bilateral carotid arteriogram and possible craniotomy. The bilateral carotid arteriorgram was normal.

B Repeat precontrast scan 10 days after the first scan shows the high density mass has resolved.

C Contrast scan reveals a very faint enhanced ring (*arrows*) that probably represents the neovasculature of the previously present perihematoma edema. This case illustrates the importance of serial scans and the merit of prudence in managing a high density mass lesion with mass effect. The patient may have a small arteriovenous malformation or a small ruptured aneurysm not demonstrated by the angiograms. The patient was still in good health on follow-up examination 3 years later.

Fig. 58. Ring-enhanced resolving hematoma 2 months after trauma in a 63-year-old woman who had fallen in the bathroom 6 days before and struck her forehead. Skull radiographs revealed a contracoup fracture in the left occiput and she was admitted with mental confusion and right homonymous hemianopsia.

A Noncontrast scan 6 days after trauma shows recent hematoma with resolution at its center.

B Repeat contrast scan 8 weeks after trauma (patient developed Jacksonian seizures on the right side) shows enhanced ring in a resolving hematoma.

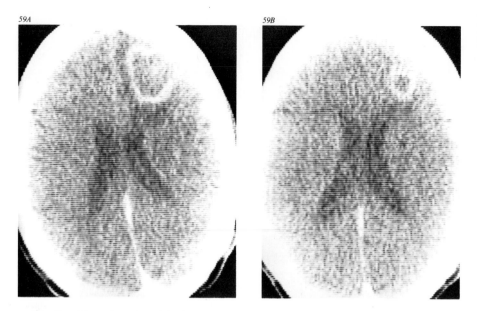

59A   59B

Fig. 61. (Right-hand page). Sequential CT in resolving hematoma with ring blush in a 66-year-old woman who was admitted with sudden onset of right hemiparesis and global aphasia. CT was performed 20 days after ictus.

A Precontrast scan demonstrates a mass lesion with high density (*arrows*), suggesting resolving hematoma.

B Postcontrast scan reveals ring-enhanced hematoma (*arrows*). It is interesting to note that there is significant mass effect and ventricular shift, even though the scan was done 20 days after the ictus. Marked ring enhancement may create confusion with other ring-enhanced lesions, such as glioblastoma multiforme and abscess.

C Repeat CT 20 days after the first scan and now 40 days after the ictus shows a marked decrease in the mass effect and in the size and enhancement of the ring blush.

Fig. 59. Ring-enhanced resolving hematoma 1 month after trauma in a 75-year-old man who had a fall 3–4 weeks ago. He was admitted with a personality change over 3 weeks, impaired memory, confusion, and bizarre behavior. The radionuclide scan showed a class IV lesion in the left frontal lobe.

A Contrast scan 3–4 weeks after trauma shows a ring-enhanced lesion with periofocal edema. Malignancy was suspected. The left carotid arteriogram revealed only a mass effect without malignant neovasculature.

B Repeat contrast scan 1 month after first CT demonstrated a marked decrease in the size of the enhanced ring and no perifocal edema. Follow-up examination 5 months later revealed no evidence of malignancy.

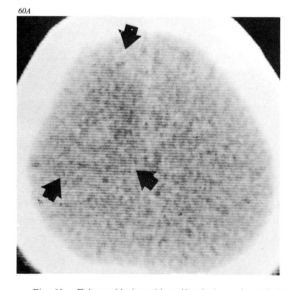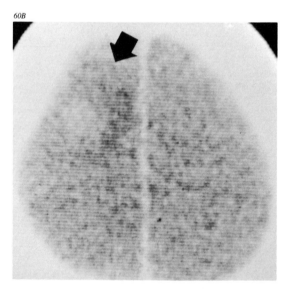

60A   60B

Fig. 60. Enhanced lesion with perifocal edema almost led to surgery, which was averted by repeat scans, in a 28-year-old man who was admitted from the emergency room because of a tonic-clonic seizure. He stated that for the last 3–4 weeks he had noticed a "funny" sensation over the left side of his body, with occasional weakness. He denied any recent trauma. Electroencephalography showed dysfunction in the right frontotemporal area and a brain scan revealed class IV astrocytoma of the right parietal lobe.

A Precontrast scan reveals an area of low attenuation (*arrows*) in the right frontoparietal region with small density in the center.

B Postcontrast scan demonstrates an enhanced discrete round lesion with surrounding edema (*arrow*). Right carotid arteriogram revealed mass effect in the right frontoparietal area. Neurosurgical consultation was obtained and craniotomy was scheduled. Repeat scan 1 day prior to surgery and 8 days after the first scan, however, revealed that the enhanced mass was considerably reduced in size. Follow-up scans revealed complete disappearance of the mass, and the patient was discharged without unnecessary surgery. This case illustrates the value of repeat scan and the nonspecificity of CT findings in enhanced masses. In retrospect, it is felt that the patient probably had a resolving hematoma or infarct.

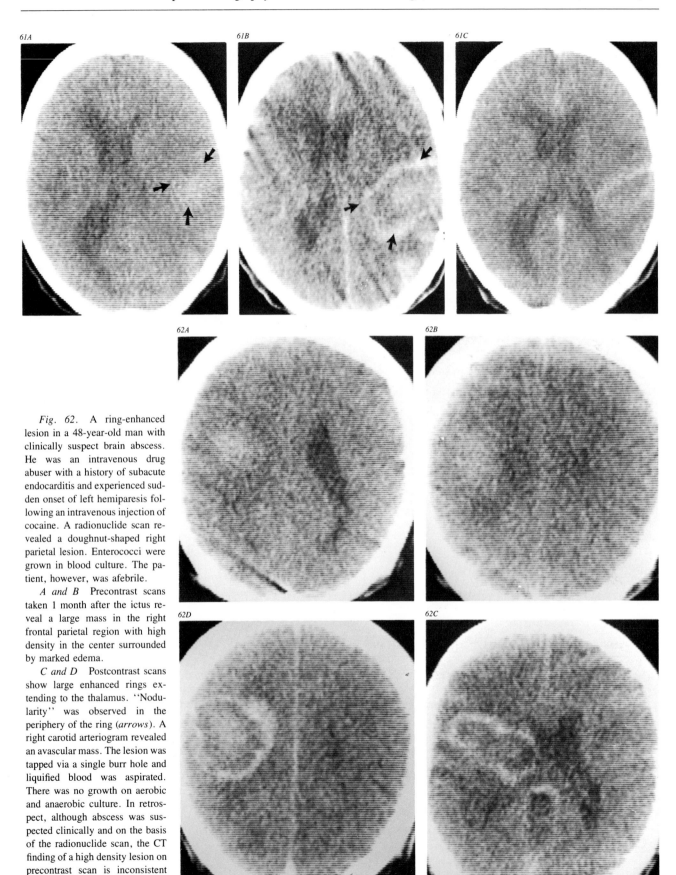

Fig. 62. A ring-enhanced lesion in a 48-year-old man with clinically suspect brain abscess. He was an intravenous drug abuser with a history of subacute endocarditis and experienced sudden onset of left hemiparesis following an intravenous injection of cocaine. A radionuclide scan revealed a doughnut-shaped right parietal lesion. Enterococci were grown in blood culture. The patient, however, was afebrile.

A and B Precontrast scans taken 1 month after the ictus reveal a large mass in the right frontal parietal region with high density in the center surrounded by marked edema.

C and D Postcontrast scans show large enhanced rings extending to the thalamus. "Nodularity" was observed in the periphery of the ring (*arrows*). A right carotid arteriogram revealed an avascular mass. The lesion was tapped via a single burr hole and liquified blood was aspirated. There was no growth on aerobic and anaerobic culture. In retrospect, although abscess was suspected clinically and on the basis of the radionuclide scan, the CT finding of a high density lesion on precontrast scan is inconsistent with abscess.

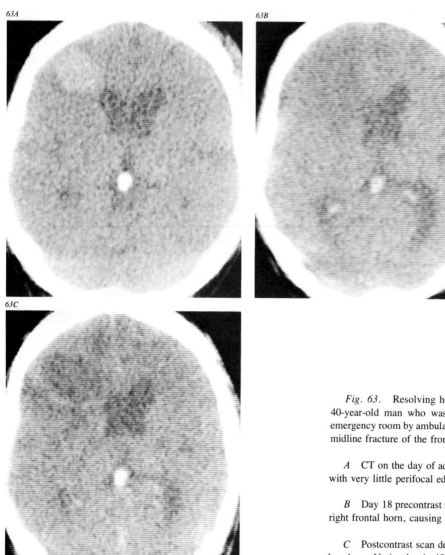

Fig. 63. Resolving hematoma with an increase in mass effect in a 40-year-old man who was found on subway stairs and brought to the emergency room by ambulance. Radiographs of his skull revealed a sagittal midline fracture of the frontal bone.

A CT on the day of admission shows a right frontal acute hematoma with very little perifocal edema and almost no mass effect.

B Day 18 precontrast scan shows low density lesion compressing the right frontal horn, causing contralateral shift of the ventricles.

C Postcontrast scan demonstrates a ring-enhanced lesion surrounded by edema. Notice the significant increase in mass effect and ventricular shift compared with the initial scan. As the patient was asymptomatic, oriented, and alert, he was discharged.

vasation of contrast agent. Consequently, CT after a contrast agent, results in a ring-enhanced appearance, which can also be seen in abscess formation, in primary or secondary malignant neoplasm, and in resolving infarct, since the neovasculature present is similar in the latter conditions. Sequential repeat scans in 2 to 3 weeks permit differentiation in most cases.

A large hematoma may take months to heal or may lead to porencephaly. A control CT for large hematomas is necessary to assess the development of porencephaly or complete resolution (figs. 64 and 65).

Intraventricular Neonatal Hemorrhage

Spontaneous neonatal intraventricular hemorrhage is a phenomenon that occurs in premature neonates. It originates in the subependymal germinal matrix, a structure located beneath the ependymal lining of the ventricles. It is a very vascular and fragile structure with little supporting tissue. The germinal matrix is largest at 24–32 weeks gestation and then involutes so that it is much smaller in full-term infants than in prematures (*Burnstein et al. 1979*). The exact cause of the hemorrhage is unknown, but contributing factors are asphyxia, the method of delivery, and the respiratory distress syndrome.

Infants with intraventricular hemorrhage usually die, or they survive with a severe neurologic handicap. CT demonstrates the location, extent, and the evolution of the intraventricular and intracerebral hemorrhage (fig. 66). It may also be used to detect the early development of hydrocephalus. According to *Burnstein et al. (1979)*, of the 22 infants

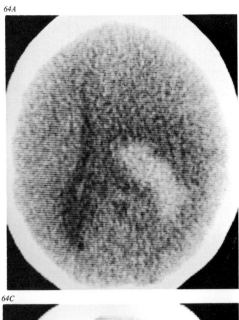

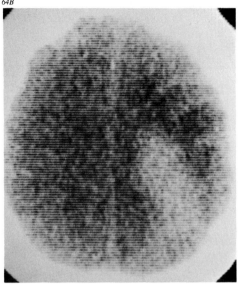

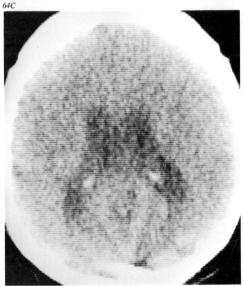

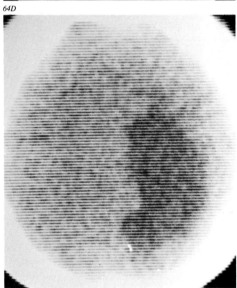

Fig. 64. Hematoma resulting in poerencephaly in a 53-year-old woman who, 12 days earlier, had subarachnoid hemorrhage with right hemiparesis. An angiogram revealed a 4 × 5 mm, left middle cerebral aneurysm at the trifurcation with a large avascular mass effect in the left high parietal area.

A and B Noncontrast scans show acute hematoma above the left lateral ventricle with perihematoma edema. Some blood is noted in the interhemispheric fissure. The exact route of the bleeding from the ruptured left middle cerebral aneurysm to this supraventricular area is still undetermined.

C and D Noncontrast scans 24 days after subarachnoid hemorrhage, when the patient was readmitted with right focal seizures, shows complete resolution (at least on the CT images) of hematoma and the formation of porencephaly.

who had CT-proved hemorrhages and survived the neonatal period, the diagnosis was not suspected clinically in 15 (68 percent).

Brainstem Hemorrhage

Hypertension is considered the most common cause of spontaneous brainstem hemorrhage. By definition, a 1.5-cm brainstem hemorrhage is considered massive. CT, inspite of frequent artifacts in the posterior fossa, can detect massive pontine and brainstem hemorrhage without difficulty (fig. 67). The prognosis of brainstem hemorrhage is far better than what was estimated in the pre-CT era. *Dhopesh et al. (1980)* reported eight cases of "primary" brainstem hemorrhage. All of their patients survived with variable recovery, except one who died of pulmonary embolus.

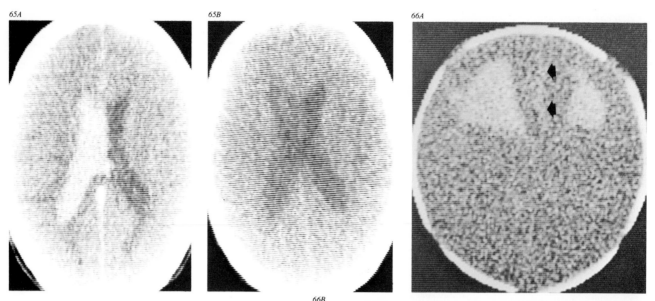

65A   *65B*   *66A*

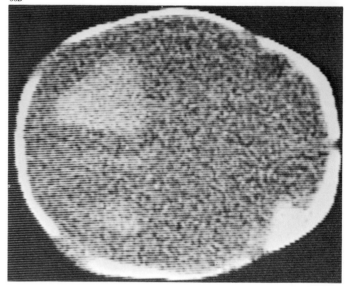

66B

Fig. 65. A 58-year-old woman presented with subarachnoid hemorrhage. From her history, it was difficult to determine whether the subarachnoid hemorrhage was spontaneous or secondary to head trauma.

A Contrast scan demonstrates acute hematoma in the right lateral ventricle.

B Repeat noncontrast scan 3 weeks later reveals complete resolution of the hematoma. Clinically, the patient made a complete recovery.

Fig. 66. Neonatal subependymal hemorrhage in a 1600-g, 36-week-old premature male born by cesarean section for fetal distress and a maternal history of preeclampsia. The infant was on respirator for seizures at 4 hours of age.

A and B CT on day 4 reveals bilateral subependymal germinal matrix hemorrhage. Blood is also seen in the interhemispheric fissure (*arrows*). Note the position of the subependymal hemorrhage in the lateral decubitus position. The findings were confirmed 2 days later by autopsy.

67

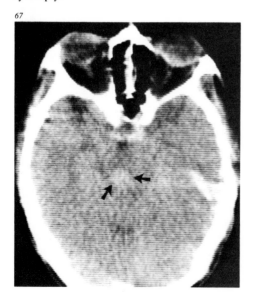

Fig. 67. Spontaneous brainstem hemorrhage in a 73-year-old woman with a history of rheumatic heart disease, mitral stenosis, and mitral insufficiency. At 1 PM she complained her right eye was blurred. She rose from her chair but sat down immediately, complaining of lack of sensation of her entire left side. Between 1 and 4 PM she had repeated projectile vomiting. Her husband noted the onset of right facial drooping and dysarthria. On admission, the patient was comatose but responded to pain. There was bilateral Babinski, right facial palsy, and absence of corneal reflexes. The noncontrast scan reveals fresh hematoma in the midbrain (*arrows*) anterior to the quadrigeminal cistern. In lower cuts (not shown) the hematoma extends down to the pons. The patient died 5 days after admission.

Arteriovenous Malformation

In the noncontrast scan, nonhomogeneous areas of increased, normal, and low tissue densities are seen. Increased tissue density is due to deposits of hemosiderin from extravasation or mural thrombus. Calcifications in the walls of the angiomatous vessels, in the draining veins, or in the parenchyma may also contribute to the high attenuation value of the arteriovenous malformation on CT. The low tissue density seen on CT is due to focal atrophy or cystic changes secondary to the malformation.

The abnormality seen on precontrast CT may be very subtle and therefore may be missed, unless the CT image is studied with extreme care (figs. 68 and 69).

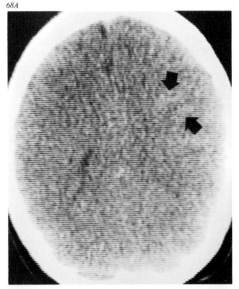

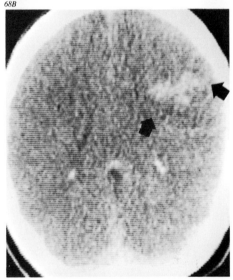

Fig. 68 A large, left frontoparietal AVM in a 42-year-old man.

A Precontrast scan shows a very subtle increase in tissue density (*arrows*) in the frontoparietal area.

B Postcontrast scan demonstrates marked irregular enhancement with small cystic areas in the surrounding area (*arrows*). The appearance of the vessels varies greatly. Depending on the angle of the cut, they may be tubular, nodular, oval, round, or curvilinear.

Fig. 69. Thalamic arteriovenous malformation draining into the vein of Galen.

A Precontrast scan shows focal dilatation of the lateral ventricle. A small cystic area is also noted (*arrow*).

B Postcontrast scan reveals tubular and curvilinear enhancement (*arrows*) in the thalamic area. The arteriovenous malformation drains into a markedly dilated vein of Galen (*arrowhead*). CT does not reveal the exact arterial supply, venous drainage, and vascular anatomy of the malformation. Arteriography is indispensable in this regard.

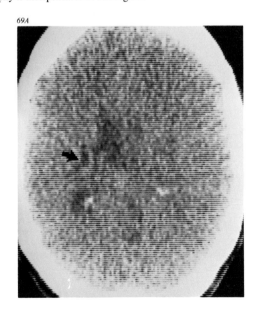

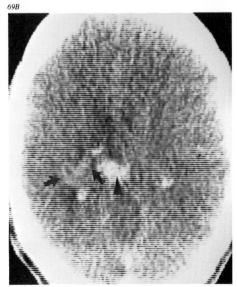

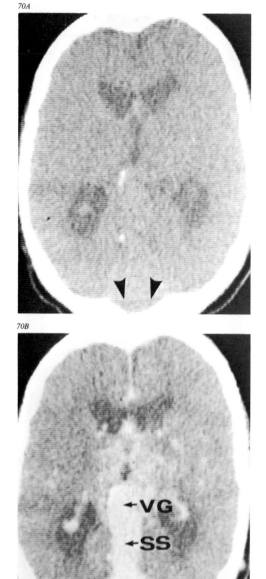

70A

70B

Aneurysm of the Vein of Galen

An *aneurysm* of the vein of Galen is a rare vascular anomaly that consists of an arteriovenous malformation and a venous aneurysm. An arterial branch may enter the dilated vein of Galen directly, or there may be a complex racemose network of noncapillary vessels interposed between the artery and vein. The postcontrast CT appearance is characterized by a large, sharply defined, enhanced vein of Galen, a straight sinus, and torcular Herophili. Prominent and irregular feeding arteries may be visible in the region of the thalami and basal ganglia bilaterally (fig. 70). The syndrome of clinically unusual congestive heart failure, hydrocephalus, and a cranial bruit in an infant should suggest an aneurysm of the vein of Galen.

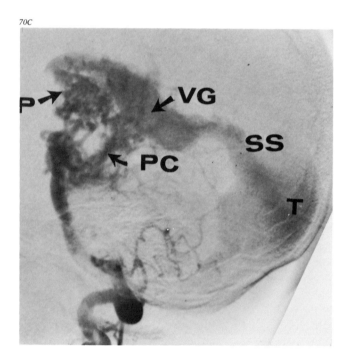

70C

Fig. 70. Aneurysm of the vein of Galen. This 12-year-old black girl was admitted because of pneumonia and congestive heart failure.

A Precontrast scan reveals an almost isodense mass lesion posterior to the third ventricle with calcifications along the right side. Depression on the inner table of the occipital bone by the enlarged torcular is noted (*arrowheads*).

B Postcontrast scan reveals marked enhancement of the vein of Galen (VG), which drains into a dilated straight sinus (SS), and torcular Herophili (T). A network of prominent feeding arteries from the thalamoperforating and choroidal branches explains the enhancement on both sides of the third ventricle.

C Vertebral arteriogram confirms the CT diagnosis. Markedly enlarged thalamoperforating branches (TP) and posterior choroidal branches (PC) are well demonstrated. Aneurysm of the vein of Galen (VG), straight sinus (SS), and torcular (T) correlate well with the CT findings.

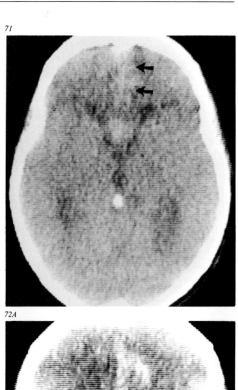

Fig. 71. Septal hematoma in a ruptured anterior communicating artery aneurysm in a 75-year-old woman with a 2-day history of cough with "cold" and a 12-hour history of persistent headache. When she was brought to the emergency room, she was lethargic, arousable, but unresponsive to verbal commands. Her neck was stiff and a lumbar puncture was grossly bloody. There were no focal neurologic signs. Noncontrast scan reveals hematoma in the septum pellucidum separating both frontal horns. Fresh blood is also seen in the interhemispheric fissure (*arrows*). On lower cuts, the blood is also noted in both Sylvian fissures and in the suprasellar cistern. The location of hematoma in the septum pellucidum is pathognomonic of a rupture of the anterior communicating artery aneurysm, which was confirmed by atuopsy in this case.

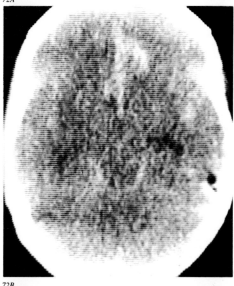

Aneurysm

Extravasated blood secondary to a ruptured aneurysm can be demonstrated by CT in more than 50 percent of cases, if the examination is performed within 5 days after a subarachnoid hemorrhage. After this period, CT usually fails to demonstrate blood in the basal cisterns. Blood density of high CT value (averaging 40 to 100 HU) can be detected in the basal cisterns, the brain parenchyma, and the ventricular system. There is no strict correlation between the distribution of blood in the cisterns and the site of the ruptured aneurysm. Blood in the interhemispheric fissure could be found in all cases of aneurysms of the anterior cerebral artery; but it could also be seen in middle cerebral aneurysms. Blood in the Sylvian fissure could be seen in a carotid syphon aneurysm and an anterior cerebral aneurysm, in addition to a middle cerebral aneurysm (*Liliequist et al. 1977*). Septal hematoma is almost pathognomonic for an anterior communicating aneurysm (fig. 71 and 72).

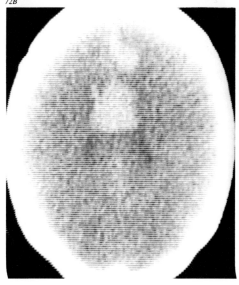

Fig. 72. Anterior communicating aneurysm ruptured into the subarachnoid space and corpus callosum of a 48-year-old woman. She had come to the emergency room with sudden severe headache, then rapidly deteriorated to stupor and respiratory arrest. Lumbar puncture yielded grossly bloody cerebrospinal fluid. She expired on day 6. Noncontrast scan on day 1 reveals:

A Blood in the interhemispheric fissure, left frontal lobe, both Sylvian fissures, and cisterns around the brain stem; and

B Hematoma in the genu of the corpus callosum, the medial longitudinal fissure extending into the left frontal lobe.

73A

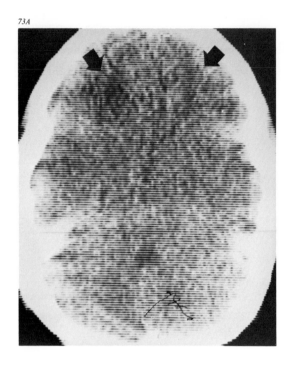

73B

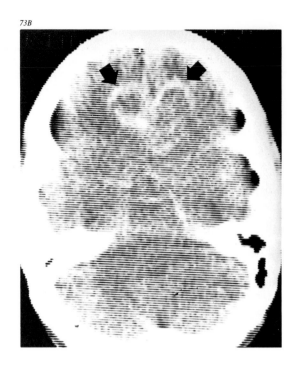

73C

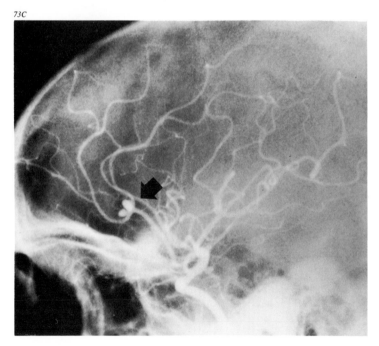

Fig. 73. Resolving hematoma with enhancing rings secondary to bilobed aneurysm in a 43-year-old woman who was admitted for bizarre behavior and class IV radionuclide scan with lesion in the left frontal lobe.

A Noncontrast scan demonstrates ill-defined low density areas in both frontal lobes, more on the right *(arrows)*.

B Contrast scan shows bilateral ring-enhanced lesions in the frontal lobes *(arrows)*.

C Bilateral carotid arteriograms reveal bilobed aneurysm arising from the A-2 segment of the anterior cerebral artery *(arrow)*. Most likely the enhanced rings represent enhanced resolving hematoma or infarction.

The extent of ischemic infarct secondary to vascular spasm in ruptured aneurysm can better be evaluated by CT than by angiography (fig. 73). Serial CT scans serve to detect the development of communicating hydrocephalus, which occurs quite frequently after subarachnoid hemorrhage.

In the past year, we have seen three cases of mycotic aneurysm with enhanced rings on contrast scans. CT was the first examination that suggested the need for an angiogram and the possibility of a mycotic aneurysm, because the enhanced rings are located in either the middle cerebral territory or in the periphery of the middle cerebral branch (fig. 74).

74A

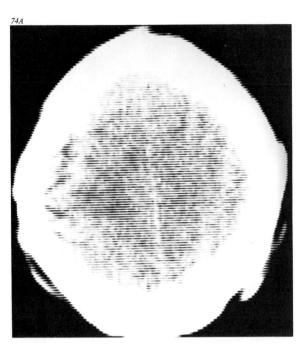

74B

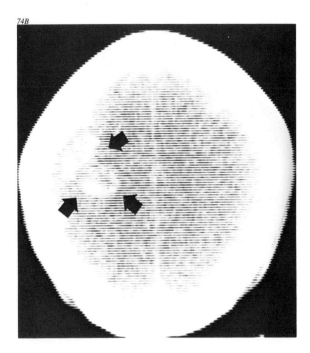

Fig. 74. Enhanced rings in mycotic aneurysm in a 23-year-old drug addict with a history of rheumatic heart disease and acute bacterial encocarditis. He had been brought to the emergency room because of high fever, seizures, increasing unresponsiveness, and left hemiparesis since the day before. The lumbar puncture was clear and contained 160 mg percent protein.

A Contrast scan 4 days after admission shows an ill-defined low density lesion in the right parietal area, degraded by motion artifacts. Emergency arteriograms were unrevealing with motion.

B Repeat contrast scan 3 weeks after the first negative scan reveals markedly enhanced rings in the right high parietal area. This precipitated a repeat angiogram.

C Repeat angiogram demonstrates a mycotic aneurysm in the middle cerebral distribution (*arrow*) surrounded by an avascular zone and luxury perfusion (*arrowheads*), which is probably responsible for the contrast-enhanced rings.

74C

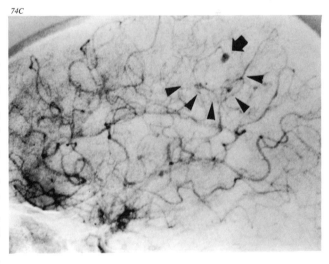

Bibliography

Albright L, Fellows R: Sequential CT scanning after neonatal intracerebral hemorrhage. AJNR 2:133, 1981.

Ambrose J: Computerized X-ray scanning of the brain. J Neurosurg 40:679, 1974.

Bell BA, Kendall BE, Symon L: Angiographically occult arteriovenous malformation of the brain. J Neurol Neurosurg Psychiatry 41:1057, 1978.

Bryan RN, Shaah CP, Hilal SK: Evaluation of subarachnoid hemorrhage and cerebral vasospasm by computed tomography. CT 3:144, 1979.

Burnstein J, Papile L, Burnstein R: Intraventricular hemorrhage and hydrocephalus in premature newborns: a prospective study with CT. AJR 132:631, 1979.

Davis JM, Davis KR, Crowell RM: Subarachnoid hemorrhage secondary to ruptured intracranial aneurysm: prognostic significance of cranial CT. Radiology 134:711, 1980.

Davis KR, New PFJ, Ojemann RG, et al: Computed tomographic evaluation of hemorrhage secondary to intracranial aneurysm. AJR 127:143, 1976.

Dhopesh VP, Greenberg JO, Cohen MM: CT in brainstem hemorrhage. J Comput Assist Tomogr 4:603, 1980.

Dolinskas CA, Bilaniuk LT, Zimmerman RA, et al: Computed tomography of intracerebral hematomas. I: Transmission CT observations on hematoma resolution. AJR 129:681, 1977.

Dolinskas CA, Bilaniuk LT, Zimmerman RA, et al: Computed tomography of intracerebral hematomas. II: Radionuclide and transmission CT studies of the perihematoma region. AJR 120:689, 1977.

Fierstien SB, Pribram HW, Hieshima G: Angiography and CT in the evaluation of cerebral venous malformations. Neuroradiology 17:137, 1979.

Gado MH, Phelps ME, Coleman RE: An extravascular component of contrast enhancement in cranial computed tomography. Radiology 117:589, 1975.

Golding R, Peatfield RC, Shawdon HH, et al: Computer tomographic features of giant intracranial aneurysms. Clin Radiol 31:41, 1980.

Grumme T, Wanksch W, Wende S: Diagnosis of spontaneous intracerebral hemorrhage by computerized tomography. In: Cranial Computerized Tomography. Edited by Lanksch W, Kazner E. Springer, Berlin, 1976, pp. 286–290.

Hayward RD: Intracranial arteriovenous malformations: observations after experience with computerized tomography. J Neurol Neurosurg Psychiatry 39:1027, 1976.

Hayward RD, O'Reilly GVA: Intracerebral hemorrhage: accuracy of computerized transverse axial scanning in predicting the underlying aetiology. Lancet I:1, 1976.

Kendall BE: CT in spontaneous intracerebral hemorrhage. Br J Radiol 51:563, 1978.

Kendall BE, Claveria LE: The use of computed axial tomography (CAT) for the diagnosis and management of intracranial angiomas. Neuroradiology 12:141, 1976.

Kendall BE, Kingsley D: The value of computerized axial tomography (CAT) in cranio-cerebral malformations. Br J Radiol 51:171, 1978.

Kendall BE, Lee BCP, Claveria E: Computerized tomography and angiography in subarachnoid hemorrhage. Br J Radiol 49:483, 1976.

Kramer RA, Wing SD: Computed tomography of angiographically occult cerebral vascular malformations. Radiology 123:649, 1977.

Krishnamoorthy KS, Shannon DC, Delong GR, et al: Neurologic sequelae in the survivors of neonatal intraventricular hemorrhage. Pediatrics 64:233, 1979.

Laster DW, Moody DM, Ball MR: Resolving intracerebral hematoma: alteration of the ''ring sign: with steroids. AJR 130:935 1978.

Lee BCP, Grassi AE, Schechner S, et al: Neonatal intraventricular hemorrhage: a serial computed tomography study. J Comput Assist Tomogr 3:483, 1979.

Liliequist B, Lindquist M, Valdimarsson E: Computed tomography and subarachnoid hemorrhage. Neuroradiology 14:21, 1977.

Lukin RR, Chambers AA, Tomsich TA: Cerebral vascular lesions: infarction, hemorrhage, aneurysm and arteriovenous malformation. Semin Roentgenol 12:77, 1977.

Martelli A, Scitti G, Harwood-Nash DC, et al: Aneurysms of the vein of Galen in children: CT and angiographic correlation. Neuroradiology 20:123, 1980.

Meese W, Aulich A, Kazner E, et al: CT findings in angiomas and aneurysms. In: Cranial Computerized Tomography. Edited by Lanksch W, Kazner E. Springer, Berlin, 1976, pp 291–297.

Messina AV, Chernik NL: Computed tomography: the ''resolving'' intracerebral hemorrhage. Radiology 118:609, 1975.

New PFJ, Scott WR: Computed Tomography of the Brain and Orbit (EMI Scanning). Williams and Wilkins, Baltimore, 1975.

Norman D: Computed tomography in intracranial hemorrhage. In: Computed Tomography. Edited by Norman D, Korobkin M, Newton TH. CV Mosby, St Louis, 1977.

O'Neill M, Hope T, Thomsen G: Giant intracranial aneurysms; diagnosis with special reference to computerized tomography. Clin Radiol 31:27, 1980.

Pressman BD, Gilbert GE, Davis DO: Computerized transverse tomography of vascular lesions of the brain. Part II: Aneurysms. AJR 124:215, 1975.

Pressman BD, Kirkwood JR, Davis DO: Computerized transverse tomography of vascular lesions of the brain. Part I: Arteriovenous malformations. AJR 124:208, 1975.

Schubiger O, Valavanis A, Hayek J: Computed tomography in cerebral aneurysms with special emphasis on giant intracranial aneurysms. J Comput Assist Tomogr 4:24, 1980.

Scott WR, New PFJ, Davis KR, et al: Computerized axial tomography of intracerebral and intraventricular hemorrhage. Radiology 112:73, 1974.

Scotti G, Ethier R, Meancon D, et al: Computed tomography in the evaluation of intracranial aneurysms and subarachnoid hemorrhage. Radiology 123:85, 1977.

Silver AJ, Pederson Jr ME, Ganti SR, et al: CT of subarachnoid hemorrhage due to ruptured aneurysm. AJNR 2:13, 1981.

Spallone A: Computed tomography in aneurysms of the vein of Galen. J Comput Assist Tomogr 3:779, 1979.

Terbrugge K, Scotti G, Ethier R, et al: Computed tomography in intracranial arteriovenous malformations. Radiology 122:703, 1977.

Weisberg L: Computed tomography in intracranial hemorrhage. Arch Neurol 36:422, 1979.

Chapter VI

Low-Grade Astrocytoma (Kernohan's Grade I and II glioma)

In most cases of grade I and II astrocytoma, noncontrast scans show decreased tissue density. As a rule, the tumors do not enhance after the injection of contrast medium (fig. 75). In only a small percentage of low-grade astrocytomas, there is slight enhancement. The presence of calcifications, would generally indicate a low-grade astrocytoma or oligodendroglioma.

Oligodendroglioma

Uniform high density calcifications with well-defined low density cystic changes are seen. Both contrast enhancement and perifocal edema are either slight or absent (fig. 76).

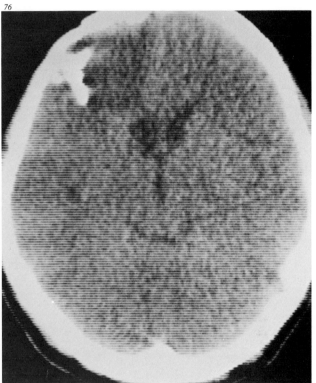

Fig. 76. Recurrent calcified oligodendroglioma with cystic changes. The right frontal horn is compressed.

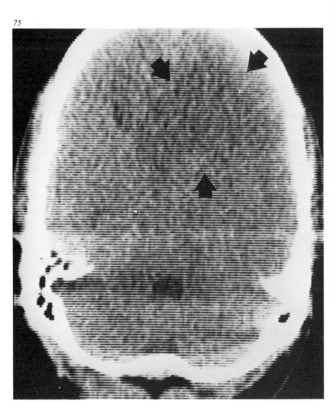

Fig. 75. Contrast scan. Nonenhanced grade IIastrocytoma in the left frontal lobe (*arrows*) with low density mass compressing the left frontal horn.

contrast scan (fig. 77). The enhancement in glioblastoma is usually quite marked; the enhanced ring is irregular, its wall either thick or thin (fig. 77). Sometimes, nodular enhancement can be detected along portions of the wall. Butterfly glioblastoma has a characteristic margin-like enhancement in the corpus callosum and ventricular wall (fig. 78).

Glioblastoma Multiforme

Also classified as grade III and grade IV astrocytoma, these tumors show density values of a mixed type on non-

Meningioma

In contrast to astrocytoma, meningioma does not show low density areas on the noncontrast scan. Indeed, most

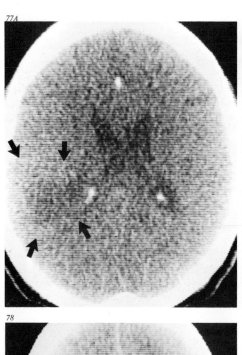

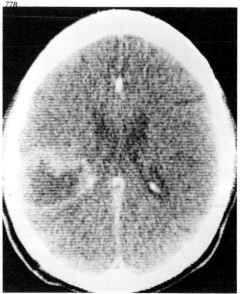

Fig. 77. Glioblastoma multiforme in the right temporal lobe.

A Precontrast scan reveals large, low density lesion surrounded by zone of faintly increased attenuation (*arrows*), causing medial displacement of the lateral ventricle.

B Postcontrast scan shows well-circumscribed but irregular enhanced annular "ring." The central lucency is probably due to necrosis. Perifocal edema is visible only on the lower sections.

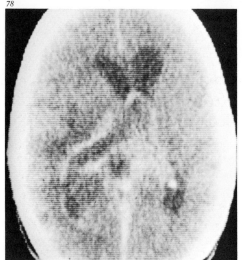

Fig. 78. Contrast scan shows enhanced butterfly glioblastoma multiforme involving the posterior corpus callosum and ventricular walls.

meningiomas have a well-defined high density or isodensity zone on plain scan study (fig. 79A). Almost all meningiomas enhance intensely and quite uniformly throughout the tumor (figs. 79B–81).

As a rule, meningioma is characterized as an homogeneously enhanced, well-defined mass located in predilection sites such as the falx, tentorium, or convexity (fig. 82). While this rule is generally correct, it is not infallible. For instance, malignant glioma or metastasis may simulate meningioma by exhibiting uniform enhancement with well-defined margins (figs. 83 and 84).

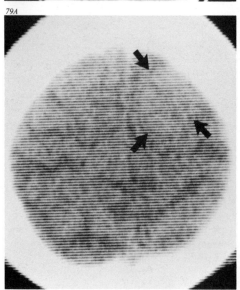

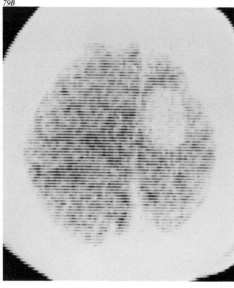

Fig. 79. Meningioma that would be missed if scans are not carried out high enough to cover the parasagittal area. The patient, a 34-year-old man, had an 8-year history of right-sided focal motor seizures.

A Precontrast scan shows a smooth, isodense mass in the left frontoparietal area, obliterating the sulci (*arrows*).

B Postcontrast scan reveals homogeneously enhanced mass (90 HU) in the left frontoparietal parasagittal area, not attached to the falx.

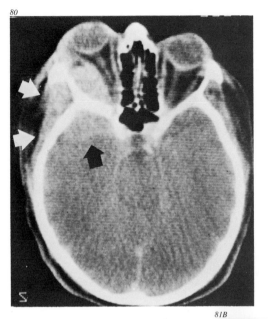

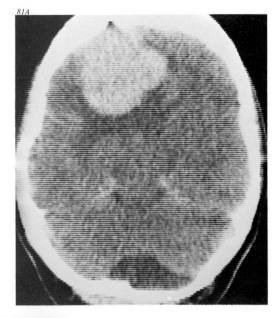

Fig. 80. Contrast scan demonstrates right sphenoid wing meningioma, which extends intraorbitally, causing medial displacement of the medial rectus, optic nerve, and exophthalmus. It also extends laterally to involve the temporal fascia and muscles (*white arrows*). Posteriorly and intracranially, it extends into the middle cranial fossa to involve the temporal lobe (*black arrow*). Note the thickened sphenoid bones, compared with the opposite normal side.

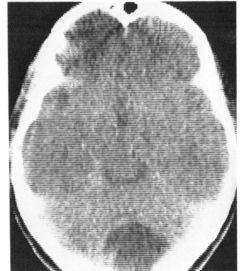

Fig. 81. Frontal convexity meningioma.

A Contrast scan reveals large enhanced meningioma arising from the frontal convexity and extending to the left side with a considerable amount of edema.

B Contrast scan 1 year postoperatively reveals total removal of the meningioma without recurrence. Large cisterna magna is noted.

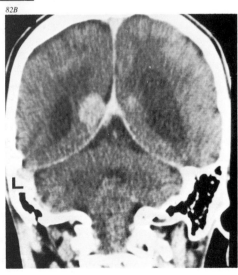

Fig. 82. A and B Postcontrast coronal scans with excellent demonstration of lobulated posterior falx meningioma, extending down to the tentorium. The lesion is noted to protrude clearly into the left trigone (*arrow*) (courtesy of Sadek L. Hilal, MD, PhD).

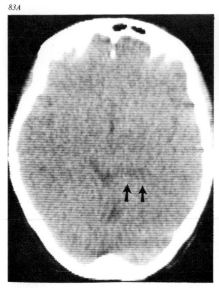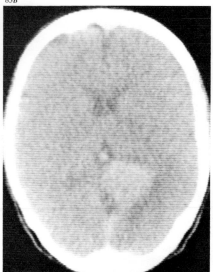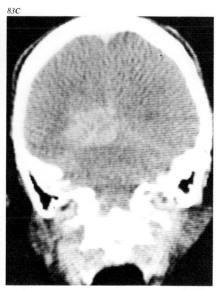

Fig. 83. This 72-year-old woman suddenly developed incoherent speech, loss of memory, and severe left frontotemporal headache. On examination she had fluent dysphasia, but no focal motor or sensory deficit. The lumbar puncture was normal.

A Precontrast scan shows grossly rotated quadrigeminal cistern, the left side being flattened (arrows).

B Postcontrast scan at a slightly higher level shows a well-defined, uniformly enhanced mass to the left side of the tentorial notch.

C Postcontrast scan in coronal plane reveals that the enhanced tumor is again well outlined, partly above and partly below the tentorium. At surgery the neoplasm was thought to have been removed almost totally and was thought to be meningioma. Pathologically, the tumor proved to be astrocytoma grade III.

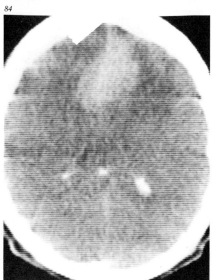

Fig. 84. Five years after a radical mastectomy for adenocarcinoma with axillary node involvement, a 66-year-old woman presented with personality change, confusion, and difficulty speaking. Contrast scan reveals a well-defined, uniformly enhanced tumor on both sides of the falx, surrounded by edema. Bilateral carotid arteriography showed an extra-axial parafalcian mass. A falx meningioma was suspected on the basis of CT finding. At surgery, metastasis to the falx was found.

In the middle cranial fossa, a small meningioma, adjacent to the petrous bone, may be associated with a large arachnoid cyst, thus leading to an erroneous diagnosis of cystic astrocytoma (fig. 85). Careful evaluation of the enhancement near the bone with proper window settings may avoid such a pitfall in interpretation.

Other atypical meningiomas such as necrotic, hemorrhagic, or cystic, are uncommon but may stimulate a malignant primary or secondary neoplasm.

A small recurrent meningioma near the base of the skull must be carefully compared with a precontrast scan to appreciate the enhancement and to distinguish the tumor from the partial volume appearance of the bony skull base (fig. 86). Overlapping scanning may be helpful.

Metastases

Four of the most common primary tumors that metastasize to the brain are bronchogenic carcinoma, breast carcinoma, malignant melanoma, and hypernephroma. About 6 percent of metastases seen on CT are solitary lesions. In two-thirds of these cases, a primary tumor is clinically evident. Perifocal edema is usually marked, while contrast enhancement is obvious and either homogeneous or ring-like in appearance (fig. 87). Differentiation from meningioma, abscess, and glioblastoma may be difficult.

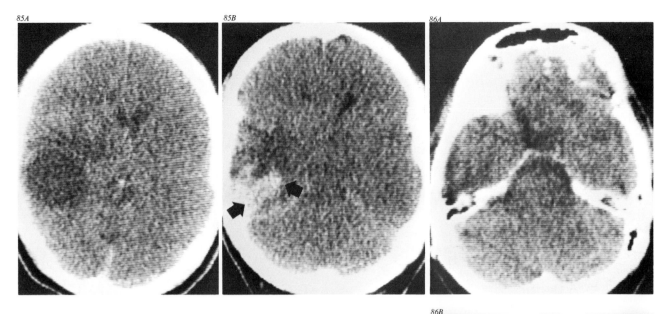

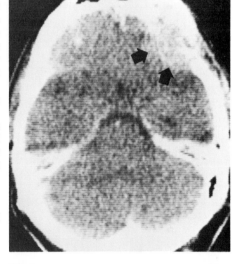

Fig. 85. Meningioma with arachnoid cyst mistaken as enhanced cystic astrocytoma in the temporal lobe, of a 56-year-old black male. He had been admitted because of the sudden onset of confusion and severe headache a day ago. In the past, he had occasional headaches, the most severe of which occurred 3 months ago. One day before admission, while at work, he again experienced a very severe bifrontal headache which was again relieved by aspirin. He got on his usual bus to go home but missed his stop and got off in a strange neighborhood where he was unable to find his way home. He could not remember his apartment location. Neurologic examination was entirely normal except for a slightly decreased left hand grip. Contrast scans showed:

A a well-defined low density, cystic lesion in the right temporal region, causing compression of the right frontal horn and contralateral ventricular shift; and

B on lower scan, some enhancement can be seen just above the tip of the right petrous bone (*arrows*). The preoperative diagnosis was enhanced cystic astrocytoma. At surgery an arachnoid cyst was seen to be capped by a very thinned-out inferior temporal gyrus cortex. As the operator looked into the cyst, he could readily visualize a tumor sitting on the floor of the middle cranial fossa, partly eroding the petrous bone. The tumor proved to be a meningioma.

Fig. 86. Recurrent left frontal convexity meningioma.

A Precontrast scan reveals evidence of a craniotomy in the left frontal region.

B Postcontrast scan shows a recurrent meningioma with homogeneous, well-demarcated enhancement (*arrows*).

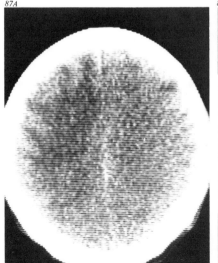

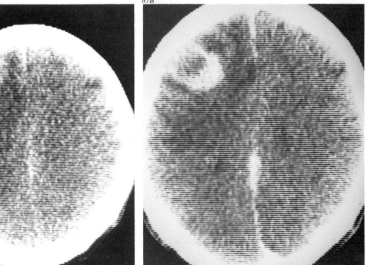

Fig. 87. Cerebral metastasis from bronchogenic carcinoma.

A Precontrast scan reveals low attenuation edema in the right frontoparietal lobe.

B Postcontrast scan shows intense annular enhancement surrounded by edema.

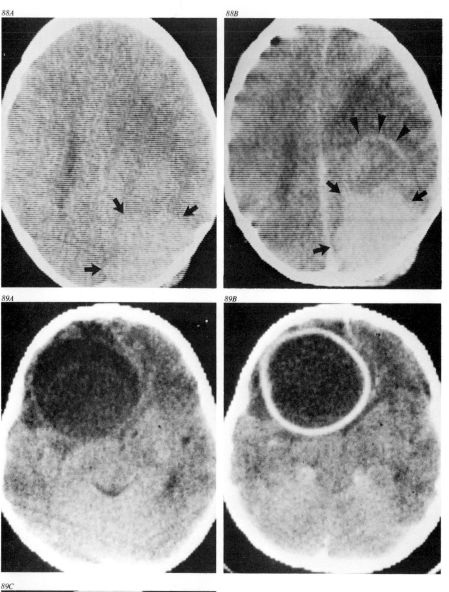

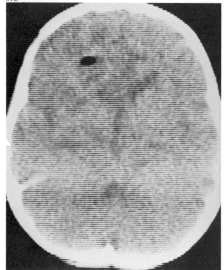

Fig. 88. Lymphocytic leukemia with intra- and extracranial metastasis in a 9-year-old boy with known acute lymphocytic leukemia. The patient had intractable headache for 3 days, markedly xanthochromic cerebrospinal fluid on lumbar puncture, and wide separation of cranial sutures. A 4 × 5 cm, firm mass was palpable in the left posterior occipital region.

A Precontrast scan shows large high attenuation mass in the left occipitoparietal lobe (*arrows*) surrounded by edema. The left lateral ventricle is compressed. The absorption coefficient in some areas measured 60–70 HU, which may represent recent hemorrhage in the metastatic lesion.

B Postcontrast scan shows markedly enhanced tumor (*arrows*) with capsular enhancement (*arrowheads*). Enhanced extracranial metastasis is also noted. Bone erosion can be appreciated on wide window setting (not shown here), but routine skull series is negative. The cerebral falx is deviated to the right side.

Fig. 89. Large frontal lobe abscess successfully drained with follow-up CT, in a 9-year-old boy from Guiana. The patient was hospitalized for an abscess of the right eyelid 7 months ago, and the abscess was drained. He subsequently developed headache, vomiting, and was hospitalized again for 40 days, but his symptoms persisted. He was transferred to St. Luke's Hospital Center in New York City. Examination there revealed mild chronic papilledema but no focal neurologic signs.

A Precontrast scan shows large, round low attenuation area in the right frontal lobe with surrounding edema.

B Postcontrast scan reveals marked enhancement of the capsule of the abscess. The enhancement of both its inner and outer wall is extremely smooth.

C Repeat scan after aspiration of 75 ml pus (Acinetobacter gram-negative cocci). A small amount of residual air is visible in the markedly shrunken abscess cavity, with a decrease in surrounding edema.

Occasionally, hemorrhage within a primary or secondary tumor can be demonstrated as a high attenuation lesion on the precontrast scan (fig. 88).

Brain Abscess and its Differential Diagnosis

On the precontrast scan, the brain abscess appears as an area of low attenuation with or without the suggestion of a rim of higher density (fig. 89A). The postcontrast scan is indispensable in diagnosing brain abscess, since almost all cerebral abscesses show ring enhancement with capsular stain, perifocal edema, and mass effect (fig. 89B and C). CT is superior to angiography, which demonstrates opacification of the abscess capsule in only 20 percent of the cases.

However, the capsular stain in an abscess, as seen on CT, is not pathognomonic; similar ring enhancement has been observed in glioblastoma multiforme, metastasis, infarction, and resolving hematoma. In malignant neoplasm, the enhanced ring is usually thicker, more irregular, and sometimes nodular. Its central zone, in the precontrast scan, often reveals some areas of high density, while it is usually of low attenuation in an abscess.

Improvement in computer software allows one to evaluate density distribution inside a pathologic zone (histogram analysis). The mean density within a lesion of interest, as measured by the cursor, is not sufficient to evaluate the nature of the lesion. Histographic analysis within a specified zone may provide information for the differentiation of various enhanced lesions, such as malignant glioma and abscess (fig. 90).

Abscesses are often multiloculate or multiple. Such information, as supplied by CT but not by angiography, is important prior to surgery (fig. 91).

Fig. 90. Compare the histogram of a glioblastoma multiforme (*A*) with that of an abscess (*B*). Note that in the tumor (*A*) the width of the histogram, the second peak, and the heterogenicity are quite different from that of an abscess (*B*).

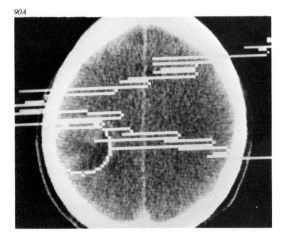
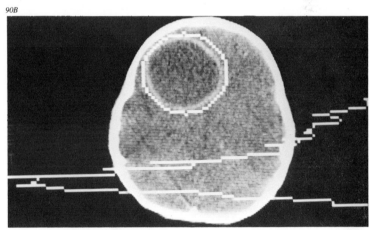

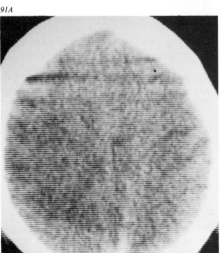
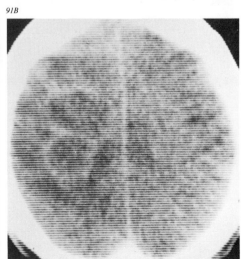

Fig. 91. Two adjacent abscesses with separate capsules. A 48-year-old man was admitted with a 1-week history of left hemiparesis.

A Precontrast scan reveals low density area in the right posterior frontoparietal region.

B Postcontrast scan shows well-defined, enhanced capsules of two abscesses with surrounding edema.

Follow-up studies are essential for the evaluation of therapeutic success. In a clinically favorable setting, some abscesses have been successfully treated without surgery (fig. 92).

Intracranial Dermoid Cyst

Intracranial dermoid cysts are rare but interesting congenital tumors. Both dermoid and epidermoid cysts derive from the displaced embryonic cells of the germinal layers, but while the dermoid cysts contain histologically hetero-

geneous materials, including desquamated epithelial cells, sebaceous products, and hair follicles, the epidermoid cysts are filled with epithelial debris and cholesterin crystals.

The dermoid cysts grow slowly and attain a considerable size without producing focal neurologic signs. Patients usually have a long history of symptoms, including headache, seizure, dementia, and meningitis.

The predilection sites of the tumors are the medial-frontobasal, juxtasellar and infratentorial regions (fig. 93). The dermoid cyst has a very high lipid content, which exceeds that of epidermoid. There is also a wide range of low densities within the cyst presumably due to its heterogeneous content. These features of a dermoid cyst make the CT appearance practically pathognomonic. The attenuation values within the dermoid cysts range between -80 and -250 HU. Although the epidermoids are also hypodense lesions, their attenuation values are rarely below -20 HU.

The cyst may erode the adjacent bones or may spontaneously rupture into the ventricle. The fat thus floating on top of the cerebrospinal fluid within the ventricle creates a fat-CSF level. While intraventricular air may give a similar appearance and a low density fluid level, the absence of preexisting cranial trauma, surgery, or spinal puncture should readily differentiate these conditions from intracranial dermoid cysts. Moreover, the absorption value of air is -1000 HU, far below that of a dermoid cyst.

Acute clinical symptoms may sometimes result from the spontaneous rupture of lipid into the ventricle and subarachnoid space, or from a meningeal reaction or vasoreactive response caused by the lipid discharged from the cyst.

Pineal Body Tumors

Management of a tumor in the region of the pineal body has undergone certain changes in recent years. Advanced microsurgical techniques have made tissue biopsy possible,

92A

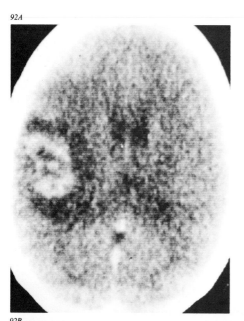

92B

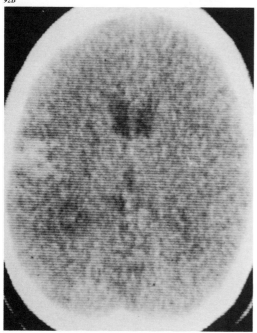

Fig. 92. Follow-up scans in a resolving tuberculous abscess in a 27-year-old Puerto Rican female who had been admitted with fever of 105° F, headache, and altered consciousness, preceded by 2 months of cough. Admission CT was normal. During the course of treatment, the patient's mental status deteriorated with the development of left hemiparesis, nystagmus, and anisocoria. Cerebrospinal fluid revealed increased protein, from 168 to 402 mg, and pleocytosis, mostly lymphocytes. Culture from the sputum for tubercle bacilli was positive.

A Contrast scan 17 days after the first negative admission scan showed an enhanced thick wall, surrounded by edema, in the abscess cavity in the right temporal lobe. The patient was treated with multiple antibiotics, steroids, and vigorous antituberculous therapy.

B Contrast scan 3 weeks later when the patient was afebrile and considerably improved shows marked reduction of enhancement and edema. The patient was followed in clinic 1 month later, at which time she had no neurologic symptoms and signs. This case illustrates the value of follow-up CT studies of patients with cerebral abscesses, which guide medical management with ultimate success.

Table 1. Classification of Pineal Tumors[a]

I. Tumors of germ cell origin
  1. Teratoma
  2. Germinoma ("pinealoma," atypical pineal teratoma, suprasellar
     germinoma, "ectopic pinealoma")
  3. Embryonal cell carcinoma (endodermal sinus tumor)
  4. Choriocarcinoma
II. Tumors of pineal cell origin
  1. Pineocytoma
  2. Pineoblastoma
III. Other cell origin
  1. Glioma
  2. Ganglioneuroma and ganglioglioma

[a] From Russell DS, Rubinstein LJ: Pathology of Tumors of the Nervous System. Fourth edition. Williams and Wilkins, 1977, pp 263–298.

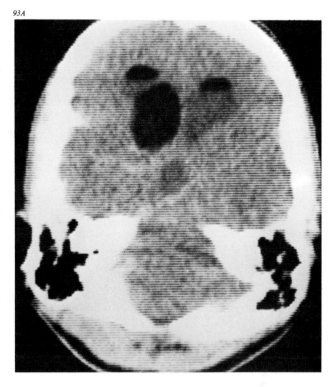

93A

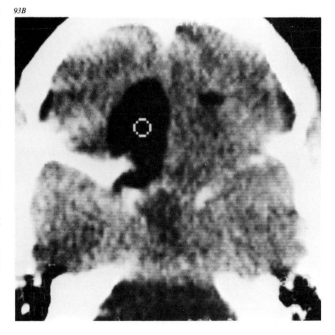

93B

and thus, more specific histologic diagnosis. It is no longer adequate to simply classify all tumors in this region as "pinealomas." Instead the Russell-Rubenstein classification has been widely accepted (see table 1).

The symptoms and physical findings are caused by obstruction of the aqueduct of Sylvius, which leads to increased intracranial pressure with headache, nausea, vomiting, and papilledema. Pressure on the superior colliculi results in loss of upward conjugate deviation of the eyes (Parinaud syndrome) and abnormal pupillary reflexes. Posterior extension of the tumor results in loss of downward conjugate deviation of the eyes, hearing impairment, and cerebellar signs, such as a positive Romberg sign, nystagmus, and varying degrees of ataxia. Inferior and anterior extension into the hypothalamus and midbrain are indicated by hypersomnia and diabetes insipidus. Certain patients have delayed gonadal function, while others have shown precocious puberty.

The treatment consists of decompression for increased intracranial pressure by ventriculocisternostomy followed by whole-brain irradiation with spinal irradiation.

In most tumors of the pineal body, CT reveals significant contrast enhancement (fig. 94). Abnormal parenchymal calcifications as well as the appearance of the quadrigeminal cistern and posterior third ventricle should be scrutinized very carefully. CT serves as a rapid noninvasive and reliable means of early detection of local recurrence and ectopic seeding to the suprasellar region.

Fig. 93. Congenital dermoid cyst in a 23-year-old woman. She had presented with a 4-year history of intermittent headache and vomiting, and the recent development of diplopia and gait abnormality. Two days prior to admission, she had episodes of hallucinations with hot flashes. Lumbar puncture at another hospital revealed increased opening pressure of 385 mm H_2O.

A and B Noncontrast scans show that the dermoid cyst has ruptured into the lateral ventricles, creating fat-CSF levels. The cursor placed on the lucent area in the right frontal region ranged from −80 to −130 HU, indicating fatty substance and other heterogeneous contents. Note the sharp bony erosion of the medial portion of the right sphenoid wing.

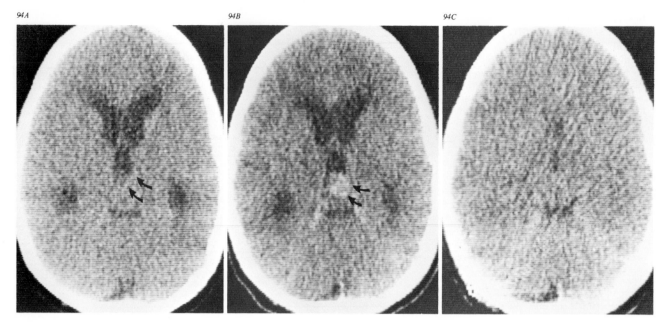

Fig. 94. Pinealoma in a 14-year-old boy who visited the emergency room three times in the past 9 months, complaining of headache, nausea, and vomiting, preceded or accompanied by fever. On examination, no neurologic signs were detected. On the last visit, the patient complained of throbbing headache over the right temporal area with intermittent vomiting. He experienced aura of scintillating lights with blurring of right vision, diagnosed as migraine. The patient's growth and development were essentially normal except for language development. On the day of admission, he presented with a 4-week history of headache, persistent vomiting, and bilateral papilledema.

A Precontrast scan reveals triventricular dilatation, including the temporal horns. Pressure effect is noted on the left side of the third ventricle (*arrows*). The quadrigeminal plate is flattened.

B Postcontrast scan shows enhanced mass protruding into the posterior third ventricle from the left side (*arrows*).

C Contrast scan 6 months after ventriculoperitoneal shunt and irradiation reveals complete disappearance of enhanced pineal tumor.

Bibliography

Aulich A, Lange S, Steinhoff H, et al: Diagnosis and follow up studies in brain abscesses using CT. In: Cranial Computerized Tomography. Edited by Lanksch W, Kazner E. Springer, Berlin, 1976, pp 366–371.

Becker A, Norman D, Wilson CB: Computerized tomography and pathological correlation in cystic meningiomas: report of two cases. J Neurosurg 50:103, 1979.

Butler AR, Horii SC, Krischeff II, et al: Computed tomography in astrocytomas. Radiology 129:433, 1978.

Butler AR, Passalaqua AM, Bernstein A, et al: Contrast enhanced CT scan and radionuclide brain scan in supratentorial gliomas. AJR 132:607, 1979.

Claveria LE, Kendall BE, du Boulay GH: Computerized axial tomography in supratentorial gliomas and metastases. In: European Seminar on Computerized Axial Tomography in Clinical Practice. Edited by du Boulay GH, Moseley IF. Springer, Berlin 1977, pp 85–93.

Claveria LE, Sutton D, Tress BM: The radiological diagnosis of meningioma, the impact of EMI scanning. Br J Radiol 50:15, 1977.

Cornell SH, Graf CJ, Dolan KD: Fat-fluid level in intracranial epidermoid cyst. AJR 128:502, 1977.

Dryer BP, Rosenbaum AE: Brain edema defined by computed tomography. J Comput Assist Tomogr 3:317, 1979.

Fawcett RA, Isherwood I: Radiodiagnosis of intracranial pearly tumours with particular reference to the value of computer tomography. Neuroradiology 11:235, 1976.

Gado, MH, Phelps ME, Coleman RE: An extravascular component of contrast emhancement in cranial computed tomography, Part I: the tissue-blood ratio of contrast enhancement. Radiology 117:589, 1975.

Gado MH, Phelps ME, Coleman RE: An extravascular component of contrast enhancement in cranial computed tomography, Part II: Contrast enhancement and the blood-tissue barrier. Radiology 117:595, 1975.

George AE, Russell EJ, Kricheff II: White matter buckling: CT sign of extraaxial intracranial mass. AJR 135:1031, 1980.

Grumme T, Steinhoff H, Wende S: Diagnosis of supratentorial tumors with computerized tomography. In: Cranial Computerized Tomography. Edited by Lanksch W, Kazner E. Springer, Berlin, 1976, pp 80–89.

Hamer J: Diagnosis by computerized tomography of intradural dermoid with spontaneous rupture of the cyst. Acta Neurochir 51:219, 1980.

Healy JF, Brahms FJ, Rosenkranz H: Dermoid cysts and their complications as manifested by computed cranial tomography. CT 4:111, 1980.

Kasner E, Wilske J, Steinhoff H, et al: Computer assisted tomography in primary malignant lymphomas of the brain. J Comput Assist Tomogr 2:125, 1978.

Lee BCP: Intracranial cysts. Radiology 130:667, 1979.

Leo JS, Pinto RS, Hulvat GF, et al: Computed tomography of arachnoid cysts. Radiology 130:675, 1979.

Lester DW, Moody DM, Ball MR: Epidermoid tumors with intraventricular and subarachnoid fat: report of two cases. AJR 128:504, 1977.

Lin JP, Kricheff II, Lagunal J, et al: Brain tumors studied by computerized tomography. In: Neoplasia in the Central Nervous System. Edited by Thompson RA, Green JR. Raven Press, New York, 1976, pp 175–199.

New PFJ, Davis KR, Ballantine HT: Computed tomography in cerebral abscess. Radiology 121:641, 1976.

New PFJ, Scott WR, Schnur JA, et al: Computed tomography with the EMI scanner in the diagnosis of primary and metastatic intracranial neoplasms. Radiology 114:75, 1975.

Paxton R, Ambrose J: The EMI scanner. A brief review of the first 650 patients. Br J Radiol 47:530, 1974.

Rao CVGK, Kishore PRS, Bartlett J, et al: CT in postoperative patients. Neuroradiology 19:257, 1980.

Russell EJ, George AE, Kricheff II, et al: Atypical computed tomographic features of intracranial meningioma. Radiology 135:673, 1980.

Russell DS, Rubinstein LJ: Pathology of Tumors of the Nervous System. Fourth edition. Williams and Wilkins, Baltimore, 1977, pp 263–298.

Steinhoff H, Lanksch W, Kazner E, et al: Computed tomography in the diagnosis and differential diagnosis of glioblastomas: a qualitative study of 295 cases. Neuroradiology 14:193, 1977.

Stevens EA, Norman D, Dramer RA, et al: Computed tomographic brain scanning in intraparenchymal pyogenic abscesses. AJR 130:111, 1978.

Sutton D, Claveria LE: Meningiomas diagnosed by scanning: a review of 100 intracranial cases. In: du Boulay GH, Moseley IF, eds: Computerized Axial Tomography in Clinical Practice. New York, Springer, Berlin, p 102, 1977.

Tadmor R, Davis KR, Roberson GH, et al: Computed tomography in primary malignant lymphoma of the brain. J Comput Assist Tomogr 2:135, 1978.

Wendling LR, Cromwell LD, Latchaw RE: Computed tomography of intracerebral leukemic masses. AJR 132:217, 1979.

Whelan MA, Hilal SK: Computed tomography as a guide in the diagnosis and follow-up of brain abscesses. Radiology 135:663, 1980.

Zimmerman RA, Bilaniuk LT, Dolinskas C: Cranial computed tomography of epidermoid and congenital fatty tumors of maldevelopmental origin. CT 3:40, 1979.

Zimmerman RA, Bilaniuk LT, Shipkin PM, et al: Evolution of cerebral abscess: correlation of clinical features with computerized tomography. AJR 127:155, 1976.

Zimmerman RA, Bilaniuk LT, Wood JH, et al: Computed tomography of pineal, parapineal, and histologically related tumors. Radiology 137:669, 1980.

Chapter VII

Sellar and Juxtasellar Lesions

For an intelligent interpretation of computed tomography in sellar and juxtasellar lesions, adequate clinical data are essential regarding pituitary function, juxtasellar cranial nerve involvement, and visual fields. The radiologist must be furnished with this information prior to the study so that additional coronal and multiple overlapping cuts with thin-section collimation may be performed and monitored after conventional scan, if a lesion becomes suspicious. Coronal sections can be achieved in a number of ways, depending on the capability of the gantry tilt, the table tilt, and the patient's capability to extend or flex the head. If the scanner's gantry can be tilted forward and backward, coronal sections can be obtained with one of the following two methods: (a) the patient is placed in the supine position, with the head fully extended (hanging-head position) and the gantry tilted 20° forward so that the plane of the scan is perpendicular to the orbitomeatal line; and (b) the patient is placed in the prone position with the head fully extended

and the gantry tilted 20° backward. If necessary, the operator may modify the degree of the gantry tilt and the patient's head position to avoid computer artifacts produced by metal fillings in teeth. Coronal sections can also be conveniently performed, if the table of the scanner can be tilted.

The coronal sections are especially useful for lesions in the region of the sella turcica, at the level of the tentorium, and in almost all areas at the base of the skull.

The most common mass lesions in the suprasellar areas are pituitary adenoma, meningioma, and craniopharyngioma. Other suprasellar lesions are chiasmal glioma, hypothalamic glioma, aneurysm, colloid cyst, ectopic pinealoma, germinoma, and epidermoid.

Pituitary Adenoma

In about three-fourths of pituitary adenomas, the density of the pituitary tumor is higher than that of the surrounding brain tissue. Suprasellar extension of the tumor is manifested by distortion and obliteration of the star-shaped suprasellar cistern. Posterior extension of the tumor can be determined by the backward displacement in the interpeduncular cistern.

Almost all pituitary adenomas reveal significant contrast enhancement of uniform density (fig. 95). Pituitary microadenoma can be detected by high resolution scanner in

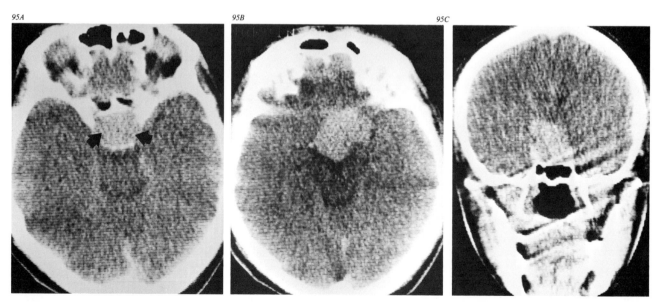

Fig. 95. Chromophobe adenoma with suprasellar extension. Contrast scans reveal:

A Markedly enlarged sella with posterior bulging of the dorsum sellae and separation of anterior clinoids. The tuberculum sellae on the left is displaced forward. Arrows point to enhanced intrasellar pituitary tumor.

B Scan above the sella demonstrate the tumor extends forward on the left side. Posteriorly the tumor displaced the interpenduncular cistern backwards.

C Coronal cut reveals upward extension of the tumor, more on the left than the right.

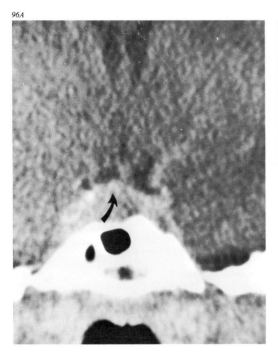

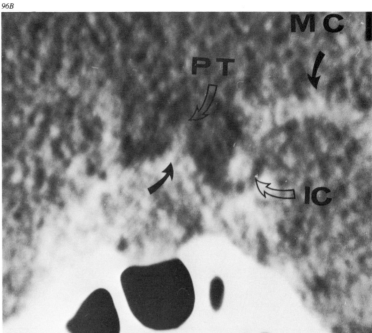

Fig. 96. Pituitary microadenoma in a 19-year-old woman with a 3-year history of amenorrhea and galactorrhea. The serum prolactin level was 270 ng/ml.

A and B Postcontrast scans at coronal planes shows the top surface of the pituitary gland microadenoma is convex upwards (*arrows*). The pitui-

tary gland is inhomogeneously enhanced, more cystic on the left side. Enhanced cavernous sinuses are seen on both sides of the pituitary fossa. The sellar floor slopes to the right side. The enhanced pituitary stalk (PT), the internal carotid arteries (IC), and the left middle cerebral artery (MC) are clearly seen (courtesy of Drs. S. R. Ganti and S. K. Hilal).

the coronal planes (fig. 96). Lesions within the sella, such as an empty sella, can also be studied best in coronal planes to avoid the partial volume effect of air in the sphenoid sinus below the sella turcica.

Meningioma

Meningiomas arising from the tuberculum sellae, planum sphenoidale, lesser wing of the sphenoid, the olfactory groove, and the diaphragm sellae, may present as a suprasellar mass. Almost all juxtasellar meningiomas show some degree of increased density on the precontrast scan and marked, uniform contrast enhancement with some peritumoral edema (figs. 97 and 98). There is no significant difference in the degree of contrast enhancement between pituitary adenomas and meningiomas (figs. 99 and 100). Even an aneurysm may present a problem in differential diagnosis. Angiography, in most cases, should be performed before surgery, not only to conclusively exclude an aneurysm, but also to provide information about the status of the vessels around the tumor, whether the vessels are encased by the tumor or merely displaced. All this information is vital for careful preoperative planning and decisions on operative approach.

A small meningioma may be missed unless appropriate angulation of the cut is obtained. Occasionally, overlapping scanning may be necessary. In studying a patient with possible recurrent meningioma, the gantry angulation may have to be altered to avoid artifacts resulting from surgical clips.

Craniopharyngioma

About half of all craniopharyngiomas are of mixed density on plain CT. Sixty to 80 percent of craniopharyngiomas exhibit some suprasellar calcifications and many of them are densely calcified. Twenty-five percent have cystic portions. Cystic tumors with calcifications are more common in children than in adults (fig. 101).

Only the solid part of the tumor can be enhanced and thus separated from the cystic parts. This very important preoperative information cannot be obtained with conventional neuroradiologic procedures. In adults, craniopharyngiomas may have to be differentiated from meningioma, pituitary adenomas, and, rarely, calcified supraclinoid aneurysms. In most cases, a careful search for a suprasellar cyst, rim calcification, and enhancement of noncystic areas are diagnostic of craniopharyngioma.

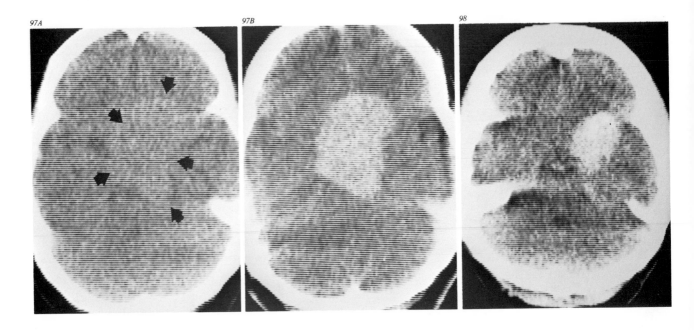

Fig. 97. Tuberculum sellae meningiona.

A Precontrast scan above the sella shows normal five-pointed star-shaped suprasellar cistern is almost completely obliterated by a large mass that is slightly denser than the surrounding brain tissue (*arrows*). A thin layer of displaced suprasellar cistern can be detected around the mass.

B Postcontrast scan at the same level shows markedly enhanced tumor with uniform density and well-demarcated borders. Arteriogram confirmed the diagnosis of meningioma and excluded the possibility of aneurysm.

Fig. 98. Left sphenoid meningioma. Contrast scan reveals markedly enhanced, well-defined meningioma arising from the lesser wing of the sphenoid. On the lower section (not shown here), bony thickening is detected on wide window setting.

Fig. 99. Parasellar meningioma in a 50-year-old man with onset of double vision 2 months ago. On examination there was left 6th nerve paralysis.

A Contrast scan reveals well-defined, homogeneously enhanced parasellar tumor.

B Coronal section reveals parasellar location of the meningioma with bony erosion of the ipsilateral sellar floor (*arrows*).

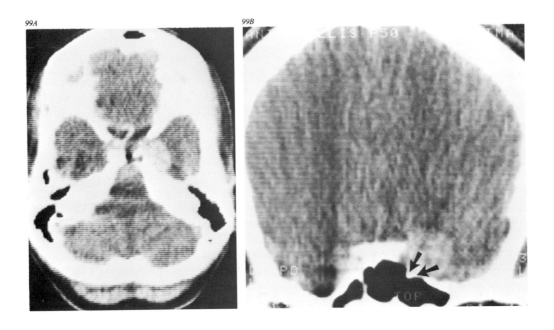

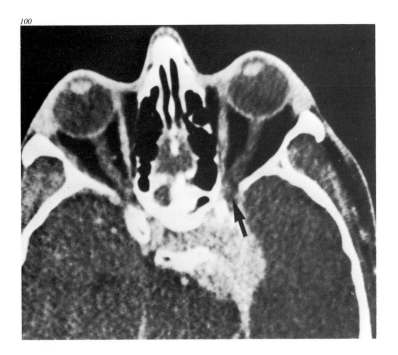

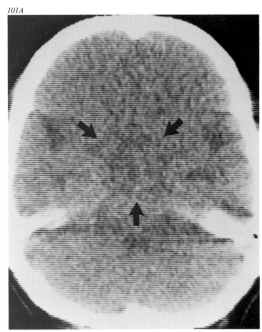

Fig. 100. Parasellar meningioma in a patient with a 4-year history of left 6th nerve palsy. The patient had numerous radiographs of the skull, the orbit, and the basal view; no lesion was detected. The present scan was performed because of the pain behind the left eye. Contrast scan reveals a large, well-marginated, uniformly enhanced meningioma in the left parasellar region of the cavernous sinus with destruction of the anterior clinoid process. The superior orbital fissure is enlarged (arrow). This case illustrates relatively little cranial nerve involvement in a large parasellar meningioma (courtesy of Dr. S.K. Hilal, MD, PhD).

Fig. 101. Cystic, rim-enhanced craniopharyngioma in a 45-year-old male with a 6-year history of visual problem and headache.

A   Precontrast scans at the suprasellar level shows large cystic mass replacing the normal star-shaped suprasellar cistern (arrows).

B   At the hypothalamic level is a cystic mass truncating both frontal horns.

C   Postcontrast scan demonstrates at the left suprasellar level, nodular enhancement on the left side (arrow).

D   Rim enhancement around the cyst.

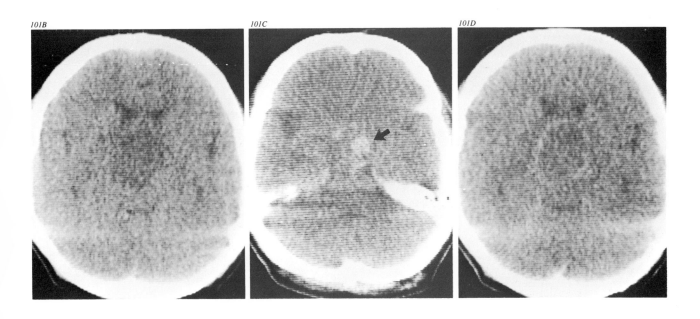

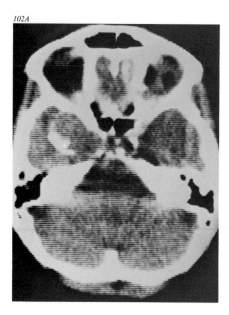

102A

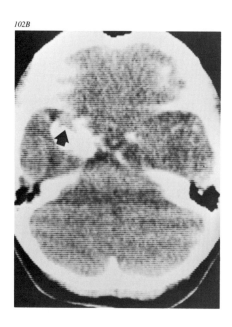

102B

Fig. 102. Large, calcified cavernous aneurysm with thrombus.

A Precontrast scan shows calcifications in the lateral wall of the aneurysm.

B Postcontrast scan reveals enhanced aneurysm in the parasellar area with thrombus (*arrow*).

C Right carotid arteriogram reveals cavernous aneurysm with thrombus (*arrow*).

Other Juxtasellar Masses

Suprasellar aneurysms may mimic pituitary adenomas and meningiomas on both pre- and postcontrast scans. The high density seen on precontrast scan may be due to intraluminal blood, mural calcification, thrombus, or a combination of these elements (fig. 102). A careful comparison of pre- and postcontrast scans can clearly identify noncalcified thrombus within the aneurysm, while angiography cannot (figs. 103 and 104). A colloid cyst of the third ventricle arises embryonically from the neuroepithelium, which is situated in the tela choroidea of the roof of the third ventricle. The lesion is located at the foramen of Monro (fig. 105). The density of a colloid cyst is usually greater than that of the brain due to ionic calcium, iron, or other organic components. The colloid cyst usually enhances after a contrast medium is administered, possibly because the radiopaque material is present in the hypertrophied choroidal vessels around the cyst, or in the cyst itself. Occasionally, a delay scan is extremely helpful for a diagnosis of colloid cyst (fig. 106). Lesions that may mimic colloid cyst include aneurysms of the tip of the basilar artery, anterior third ventricle ependymoma, astrocytoma of the third ventricle, and even craniopharygioma.

Chiasmal and optic glioma may have a very dense contrast enhancement, or none at all (fig. 107). When a chiasmal glioma reaches the hypothalamus, it is difficult to distinguish it from primary hypothalamic glioma.

Clivus chordoma and meningioma are primarily retrosellar in location, but may extend to the suprasellar region (fig. 108). Lesions below the sella, such as nasopharyngeal tumor and mucocele of the sphenoid sinus, may extend upward to invade the sella. Computed tomography, especially in the coronal planes, is extremely valuable in assessing the extent of the bony and soft tissue involvement (fig. 109).

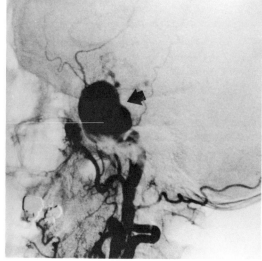

102C

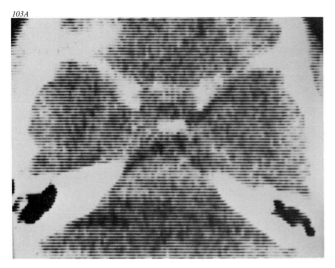

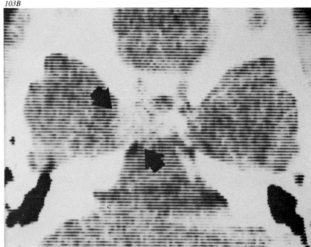

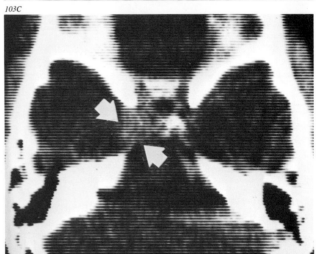

Fig. 103. Cavernous aneurysm viewed with different window width. A 55-year-old female presented with 3-month history of right retro-orbital pain, 2-week history of blurred vision, and ptosis of the right eye for 1 week.

A Precontrast scan shows no abnormality is detected.

B Postcontrast scan reveals enhanced lesion in the right parasellar area (*arrows*). Cavernous aneurysm was suspected and subsequently confirmed by angiogram.

C Same image as (*B*). View with wider window width and higher window center shows better distinction between bony sella and enhanced aneurysm (*arrows*).

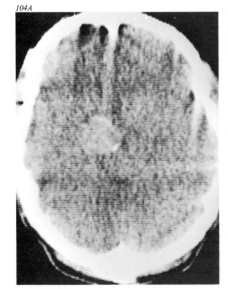

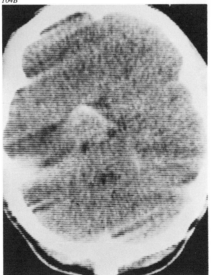

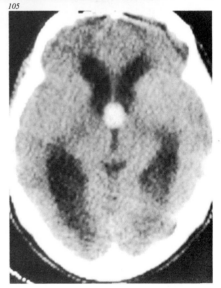

Fig. 104. Occluded giant aneurysm of the right carotid bifurcation, which was treated with common carotid ligation 7 years ago.

A Precontrast scan reveals calcified aneurysm with large mural thrombus.

B Postcontrast scan reveals occluded aneurysm with thrombus.

Fig. 105. Colloid cyst of the third ventricle. Noncontrast scan demonstrates a rounded mass with extremely high attenuation value situated at the foramen of Monro, causing obstructive hydrocephalus.

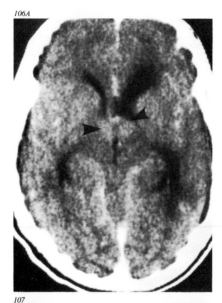
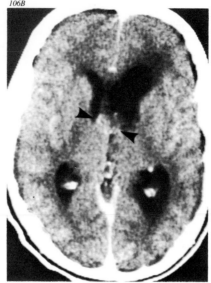
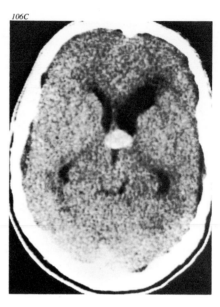

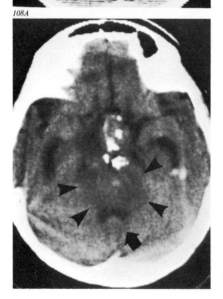

Fig. 106.   Colloid cyst in a 16-year-old boy who presented with headache and bilateral papilledema.

A Contrast scan at the level of the foramen of Monro demonstrates a rounded mass of a density close to that of the basal ganglia (*arrowheads*). The mass has a convex forward border and obliterates the anterior portion of the third ventricle. The left frontal horn is dilated due to partial obstruction of the foramen of Monro by the mass. Discernible is a septum pellucidum cyst, partly obscured by the dilated left frontal horn.

B Contrast scan at a level immediately above *A*. The wall of the mass is slightly and incompletely enhanced (*arrowheads*). While a diagnosis of colloid cyst was suspected, other possibilities such as hypothalamic glioma or thrombotic aneurysm were not entirely excluded.

C Delayed scan obtained 2 days later, without additional contrast medium, shows intense enhancement of the colloid cyst, which is slightly larger on the left side, causing partial ipsilateral blockage of the foramen of Monro. Delayed enhancement of colloid cyst, which persists for 2 days, is most unusual and has not been reported before (courtesy of Dr. LeRoy M. Kotzen).

Fig. 107   Chiasmatic glioma in a 3-year-old girl who presented with a history of frequent falls. Skull films reveal widening of sutures and enlarged sella. Contrast scan demonstrates intensely enhanced suprasellar tumor causing obstructive hydrocephalus.

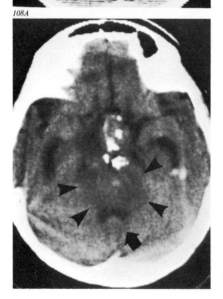
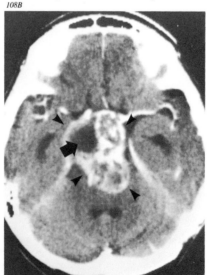
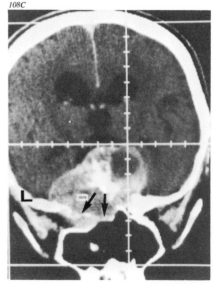

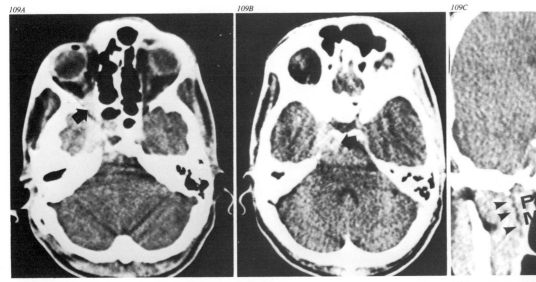

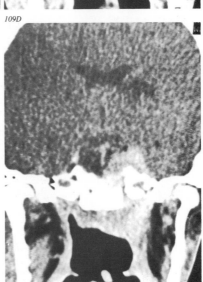

Fig. 109. Nasopharyngeal squamous cell carcinoma in a 26-year-old male, extending into the right parasellar region. The patient developed progressive right facial numbness with ptosis.

A Contrast scan in axial planes show an enhanced right parasellar mass extending into the posterior ethmoid cells and right orbital apex (*arrow*).

B Invasion of the tumor to the right prepontine cistern (*arrow*).

C Contrast scan in coronal planes shows, at the level of posterior clinoids, the parasellar soft tissue mass, which is much larger than the nasopharyngeal mass (*arrow*). Note the normal paranasopharyngeal space (*arrowheads*), intrapharyngeal muscle (PM) and patent lateral pharyngeal recess (*white arrow*) on the left.

D Scan 2 cm posteriorly reveals a much larger nasopharyngeal tumor completely obliterating the lateral pharyngeal recess and invading the lateral wall of the nasopharynx. At this level, the intracranial extension of the tumor is smaller than the nasopharyngeal mass but invades the pituitary fossa and the suprasellar cistern (courtesy of S. K. Hilal, MD, PhD).

Fig. 108. Chordoma.

A Precontrast scan shows irregular, dense calcifications in the suprasellar and retrosellar regions. No capsular rim is detected. The fourth ventricle is displaced posteriorly (*arrow*), and a large low density lesion is seen to involve the brain stem (*arrowheads*).

B Postcontrast scan shows a large, bulky, lobulated mass containing dense calcifications was demonstrated with mixed degree of enhancement. The enhanced capsule of the tumor is well-defined (*arrowheads*). The nonenhanced part (*arrow*) of the tumor is also well-delineated.

C Contrast scan in coronal plane reveals destruction of the skull base and downward extension of the tumor into the pharyngeal space (*arrows*). The enhanced mass has attenuation values of +40 HU (courtesy of Dr. W. C. Yang).

Bibliography

Bajraktari X, Bergstrom M, Brismar L, et al: Diagnosis of intrasellar cisternal herniation (empty sella) by computer assisted tomography. J Comput Assist Tomogr 1:105, 1977.

Banna M, Baker Jr HL, Houser OW: Pituitary and parapituitary tumors on CT. Br J Radiol 53:1123, 1980.

Britt RH, Silverberg GD, Enzmann DR, et al: Third ventricular choroid plexus arteriovenous malformation simulating a colloid cyst. J Neurosurg 52:246, 1980.

Byrd SE, Bentson JR, Winter J, et al: Giant intracranial aneurysms simulating brain neoplasms on computed tomography. J Computed Assist Tomogr 2:303, 1978.

Chang CH, Pool JL: Radiotherapy in pituitary adenoma. Radiology 89:1005, 1967.

Daniels DL, Haughton VM, Williams AL, et al: Computed tomography of the optic chiasm. Radiology 137:123, 1980.

Fahlbusch R, Grumme T, Aulich A, et al: Suprasellar tumors in the CT scan. In: Cranial Computerized Tomography. Edited by Lanksch W,

Kazner E. Springer, Berlin, 1976, pp 114–127.

Firooznia H, Pinto RS, Lin J, et al: Chordoma: radiologic evaluation of 20 cases. AJR 127:797, 1976.

Fitz CR, Wortzman G, Harwood-Nash DD, et al: Computed tomography in craniopharyngiomas. Radiology 127:687, 1978.

Ganti SR, Antunes JL, Louis KM, et al: Computed tomography in the diagnosis of colloid cysts of the third ventricle. Radiology 138:385, 1981.

Glydensted C, Karle A: Computed tomography of intra- and juxtasellar lesions: a radiological study of 108 cases. Neuroradiology 14:5, 1977.

Gross CE, Binet EF, Esguerra JV: Metrizamide cisternography in the evaluation of pituitary adenomas and the empty sella syndrome. J Neurosurg 50:472, 1979.

Hall K, McAllister VL: Metrizamide cisternography in pituitary and juxtapituitary lesions. Radiology 134:109, 1980.

Hammerschlag SB, Wolpert SM, Carter BL: Computed coronal tomography. Radiology 120:219, 1978.

Hatam A, Bergstroem M, Greitz T: Diagnosis of sellar and parasellar lesions by computed tomography. Neuroradiology 18:249, 1979.

Hoffman JC, Jr, Tindall GT: Diagnosis of empty sella syndrome using Amipaque cisternography combined with computed tomography. J Neurosurg 52:99, 1980.

Kendall BE, Lee BCP: Cranial chordomas. Br J Radiol 50:687, 1977.

Leeds NE, Naidich TP: Computed tomography in the diagnosis of sellar and papasellar lesions. Semin Roentgenol 12:121, 1977.

Mancuso AA, Bohnman L, Hanafee W, et al: Computed tomography of the nasopharynx: normal and variants of normal. Radiology 137:113, 1980.

Miller JH, Pena AM, Segall HD: Radiological investigation of sellar region masses in children. Radiology 134:81, 1980.

Naidich TP, Pinto RS, Kushner MJ, et al: Evaluation of sellar and parasellar masses by computed tomography. Radiology 120:91, 1976.

New PFJ, Scott WR: Computed tomography of the brain and orbit (EMI scanning). Williams and Wilkins, Baltimore, 1975.

New PFJ, Scott WR, Schnur JA, et al: Computed tomography with the EMI scanner in the diagnosis of primary and metastatic intracranial neoplasms. Radiology 114:75, 1975.

Paxton R, Ambrose J: The EMI scanner: a brief review of the first 650 patients. Br J Radiol 47:530, 1974.

Reich NE, Zelch JV, Alfridi RJ, et al: Computed tomography in the detection of juxtasellar lesions. Radiology 118:333, 1976.

Sackett JF, Messina AV, Petito CK: Computed tomography and magnification vertebral angiotomography in the diagnosis of colloid cysts of the third ventricle. Radiology 116:95, 1975.

Salvolini U, Menichelli F, Pasquini U: Sellar region: normal and pathologic conditions. In: Clinical Computer Tomography—Head and Trunk. Edited by Baert A, Jeanmart L, Wackenheim A. Springer, Berlin 1978, pp 14–37.

Savoiardo M, Harwood-Nash DC, Tedmor R, et al: Gliomas of the intracranial anterior optic pathways in children. Radiology 138:601, 1981.

Strand RD, Baker RA, Ordia IJ, et al: Metrizamide ventriculography and computed tomography in lesions about the third ventricle. Radiology 128:405, 1978.

Takeuchi J, Handa H, Otsuka S, et al: Neuroradiological aspects of suprasellar germinoma. J Neurosurg 49:41, 1978.

Wolf BS, Nakagawa H, Staulcup PH: Feasibility of coronal views in computed scanning of the head. Radiology 120:217, 1976.

Wolfmann NT, Boehnke M: The use of coronal sections in evaluating lesions of the sellar and parasellar regions. J Comput Assist Tomogr 2:308, 1978.

Detection of a posterior fossa mass is more difficult than a supratentorial mass because the territory of the former is relatively small and surrounded by dense bony structures. The petrous bones, the air in the mastoid cells, and the prominent internal occipital protuberance often result in artifacts, which are accentuated by slight motion.

The scans are made routinely with a 20°–25° tilt of the gantry against Reid's line. Occasionally overlapping and coronal cuts are used. Both pre- and postcontrast studies are necessary for complete examination, since a small lesion might not be appreciated without a precontrast image for comparison.

Motion artifacts must be reduced to a minimum, either by sedation or by general anesthesia, if necessary.

Cerebellar Metastases

Cerebellar metastasis is the most common neoplasm and mass lesion in the adult population. The precontrast scan is nonuniform in density and may be hypodense, isodense, hyperdense, or a mixture of densities. The overwhelming majority of cases show postcontrast enhancement, which may be ring-shaped, nodular, or mixed (fig. 110). Perifocal edema is usually marked. A significant number of cerebellar metastases do not cause hydrocephalus. And, the degree of hydrocephalus is related less to the size of the tumor itself than to its position and the extent of its perifocal edema.

Recent technical advances in the computer science have enabled us to reconstruct sagittal and coronal images from axial pictures, by way of computer manipulation. By de-

convoluting the data through a computer algorithm, images in sagittal and coronal planes are reconstructed. To reduce radiation exposure, *Maravilla (1978)* uses, contiguous, nonoverlapping, 3-mm thin-section scans.

Primary Posterior Fossa Neoplasms

The three most common primary neoplasms in the posterior fossa are astrocytoma, medulloblastoma, and hemangioblastoma. The mean age of patients who develop astrocytoma and medulloblastoma is under 20 years, while that for hemangioblastoma is about 48 years.

Medulloblastoma

Medulloblastoma is a common posterior fossa tumor in children, second only to cerebellar astrocytoma. The peak incidence is in the first 6 years of life. The tumor arises in the midline from the roof of the fourth ventricle, but grows anteriorly into the fourth ventricle and posteriorly and laterally to the vermis and cerebellar hemispheres. The tumor

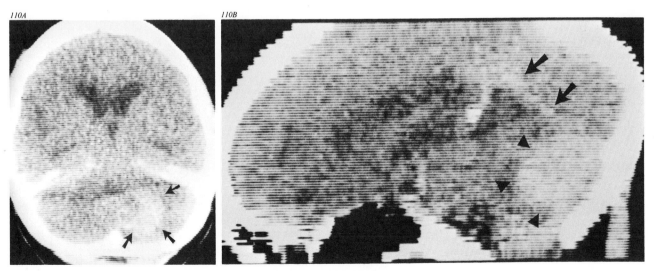

Fig. 110. Right cerebellar metastasis from bronchogenic carcinoma in a 72-year-old female with a history of resection of bronchogenic carcinoma 2 years ago.

A Contrast scan shows enhanced nodular mass (*arrows*) in the right cerebellar hemisphere. Transverse scans, 8 mm in thickness, are taken with 3 mm overlapping. The data are then reconstructed by the computer and

images in the sagittal and coronal planes are obtained.

B Reconstructed sagittal scan demonstrates the relationship between tumor (*arrowheads*) and tentorium (*arrows*), which is now clearly displayed. The tumor is shown to be entirely below the tentorium. The full vertical extent of the tumor cannot be appreciated from the transverse scans.

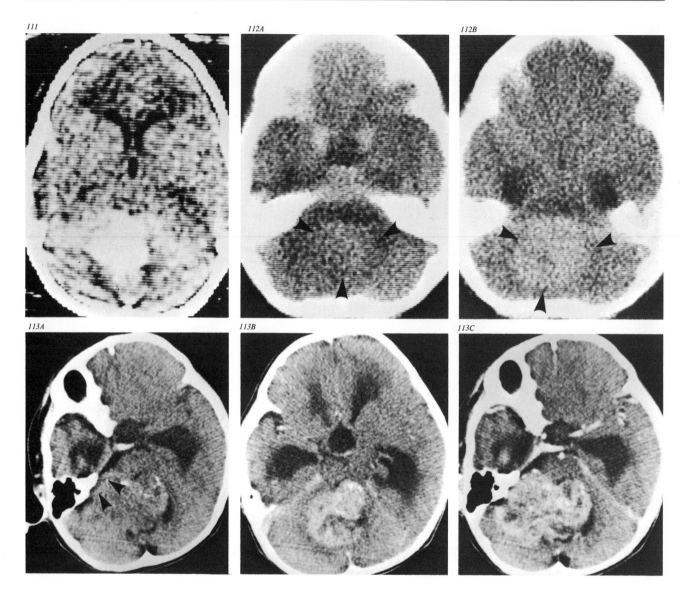

Fig. 111. Enhanced medulloblastoma in a 3-year-old girl who presented with spontaneous subarachnoid hemorrhages on two occasions, without localizing signs. Contrast scan shows the tumor has filled the entire fourth ventricle and extended laterally to the right cerebellar hemisphere. The mass is surrounded by a zone of edema. Despite the size and position of the tumor, no hydrocephalus has yet occurred.

Fig. 112. Medulloblastoma in a 3-year-old girl with supratentorial extension. The girl was born with Fanconi's anemia and left clubfoot. She presented with a history of ataxia for 4 weeks and lethargy for 2 weeks, followed by occipital headache and projectile vomiting 1 week before admission. Over the past 24 hours her mental status has changed and she is now between deep somnolence with no response to pain, and brief moments of wakefulness during which she is aware of very little.

A Precontrast scan shows a large rounded mass, of a density slightly higher than that of the brain, occupying a large part of the posterior fossa. The mass is surrounded by edema (*arrowheads*).

B Postcontrast scan reveals enhancement of the entire rounded, smoothly demarcated mass (*arrowheads*). Note the markedly dilated tem-

poral horns. The higher scans (not shown) reveal extension of the tumor into the right occipital lobe. At surgery, a huge midline medulloblastoma was resected. The tumor extended above the tentorium and has protruded into the right occipital horn. Despite a full course of irradiation to the whole brain and spinal axis, the patient died of recurrence 11 months later.

Fig. 113. Ependymoma with calcifications in a 6-month-old girl.

A Precontrast scan reveals scattered flecks of calcifications in a large lobulated soft tissue tumor, partly surrounded by cerebrospinal fluid. The tumor extends into the right cerebellopontine angle and markedly compresses its cistern (*arrowheads*). Both temporal horns and the lower third ventricle are markedly dilated.

B and C Postcontrast scans reveal a very bulky, lobulated tumor with pronounced enhancement. A part of the tumor is outlined by cerebrospinal fluid in the displaced fourth ventricle. The tumor contains numerous cystic or necrotic foci. Cerebellopontine extension is also obvious. While medulloblastoma was not conclusively excluded on CT, the bulky, calcium-containing, intrafourth ventricular tumor strongly suggested an ependymoma, which was confirmed surgically (courtesy of Drs. S. R. Ganti and S. K. Hilal).

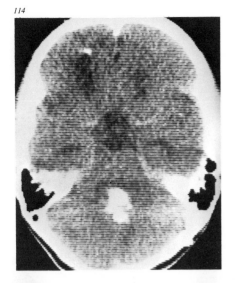

114

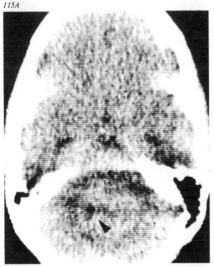

115A

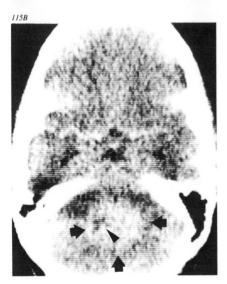

115B

Fig. 114. Recurrent calcified cystic astrocytoma in a 16-year-old female, who presented with a 2-month history of intermittent vomiting 3 years after craniotomy for cerebellar astrocytoma. The tip of a ventriculoatrial shunt catheter is seen in the right frontal horn.

Fig. 115. Hemangioblastoma.
A Precontrast scan reveals a solid tumor of brain density completely obliterating the fourth ventricle. A small cyst is noted in the right side of the tumor (*arrowhead*).
B Postcontrast scan shows marked enhancement of the tumor (arrows) with a small unenhanced cyst (*arrowhead*) (courtesy of Dr. Y. P. Huang, Mount Sinai Hospital, New York City).

is malignant and invasive and tends to seed into the cranial and spinal subarachnoid space. The post contrast scan reveals marked homogeneous enhancement with perifocal edema (figs. 111 and 112). At times, medulloblastoma may be difficult to differentiate from ependymoma of the fourth ventricle (fig. 113).

Cerebellar Astrocytoma

Cerebellar astrocytoma is the most common posterior fossa tumor in children. It is considered the most benign, and it has the best prognosis. On noncontrast scan, the typical finding is a large well-defined cyst with a small mural nodule of isodensity. The mural nodule may become densely enhanced after contrast administration. The cyst wall may also be enhanced. Occasionally, dense calcifications may be seen in astrocytomas (fig. 114).

Hemangioblastoma

Hemangioblastoma is either of cystic or mixed density on precontrast scan. Enhancement may be nodular, patchy, or ring-like. Differential diagnosis from cystic astrocytoma may occasionally present a problem. In all infratentorial tumors, posterior fossa arteriography is usually performed to assess the vascular supply, if surgery is contemplated. (figs. 115 and 116).

Brain Stem Glioma

Both primary brain stem glioma as well as metastasis may reveal obvious or very subtle backward displacement, or nonvisualization of the fourth ventricle, and compression of the pontine cistern should arouse suspicion of a pontine glioma (fig. 117). If necessary, limited pneumoencephalography may be performed prior to radiation therapy.

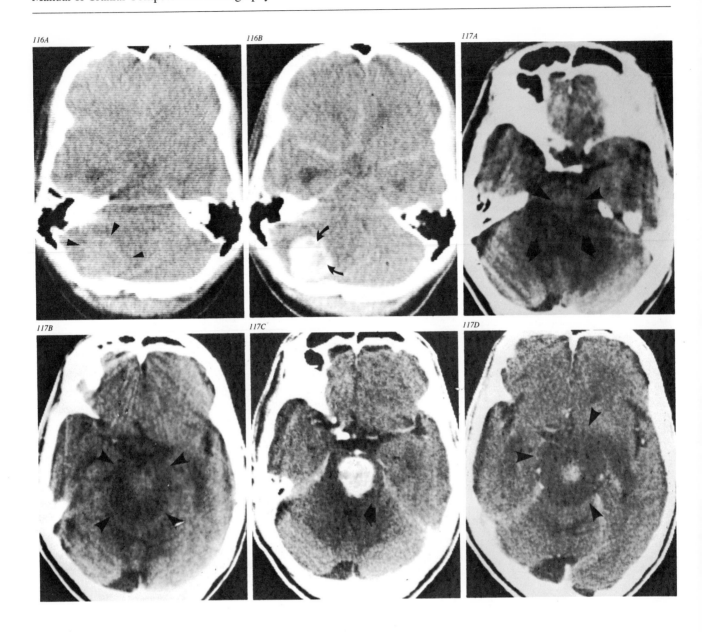

Fig. 116. Hemangioblastoma in a 34-year-old man who presented with a 6-month history of headache and 1½ month history of ataxia. On examination there was nystagmus on right lateral gaze and rotary nystagmus on upward gaze.

A Precontrast scan shows high attenuation lesion in the right cerebellar hemisphere (*arrowheads*) with perifocal edema.

B Postcontrast scan demonstrates densely enhanced tumor with two cystic lesions (*arrows*) within. There is a considerable amount of edema around the tumor, and the fourth ventricle is compressed and displaced to the left side. Both temporal horns are dilated and on higher level there is hydrocephalus. The preoperative diagnosis of hemangioblastoma was confirmed at surgery.

Fig. 117. Brain stem metastasis in a 61-year-old man with lung carcinoma. Precontrast scans show

A the fourth ventricle obscured by considerable artifacts created by the occipital protuberance, is displaced backwards (*arrows*). An oval lesion, slightly denser than the surrounding brain, is seen in the pontine region (*arrowheads*).

B The scan immediately above (A) reveals the oval-shaped high density lesion in the brain stem, surrounded by edema (*arrowheads*). The five-pointed, star-shaped suprasellar cistern is grossly distorted. Normal perimesenteric cisterns are obliterated by the edema.

C Postcontrast scans show (C intense enhancement of pontine metastatic tumor surrounded by marked edema posteriorly. Compare this image with (A). This image is slightly higher, just above the external and internal occipital protuberance, and thus avoids many radiating dense and lucent streaks produced by the computer artifacts. However, only the uppermost part of the fourth ventricle is included in this image (*arrow*), and does not appear to be displaced.

D Enhanced lesion reaches the midbrain. The edema extends forward to the thalami and obliterates the posterior third ventricle (*arrowheads*) (courtesy of Dr Wen-Chang Yang).

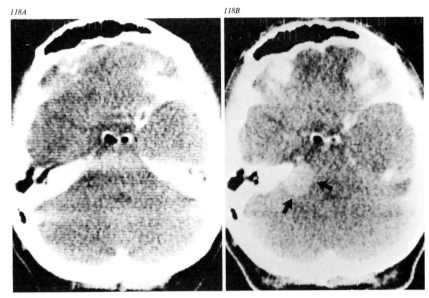

Fig. 118. Acoustic neuroma.

A Precontrast scan shows no detectable abnormality.

B Postcontrast scan shows densely enhanced, well-defined tumor in the right cerebellopontine angle (*arrows*).

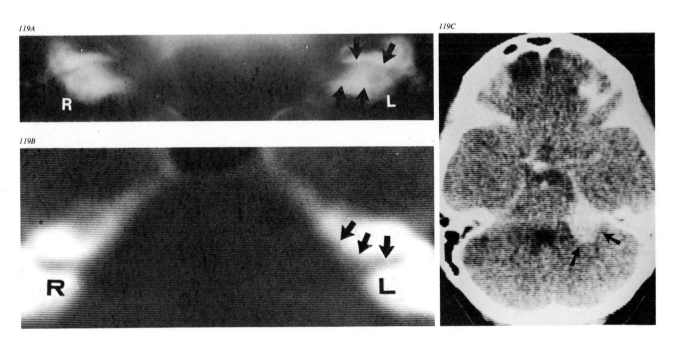

Cerebellopontine Angle Lesions

Acoustic neuroma is the most common cerebellopontine angle neoplasm, comprising about 75 percent of neoplasms in that area (figs. 118 and 119). Meningiomas, epidermoids (cholesteatomas), metastases, aneurysms, and glomus jugulare tumors have been found in the cerebellopontine angle area (figs. 120 and 121). Acoustic neuroma can be detected by CT in about only 75 percent of the cases, even with the overlapping technique, both with and without contrast administration. Most neuromas appear isodense or hypodense on precontrast scan but become markedly hyperdense after enhancement.

Fig. 119. Acoustic neuroma with normal polytomograph from a 61-year-old female who presented with a 5-year history of progressive hearing loss of the left ear and burning sensation of the tongue and face on the left side in recent months. Polytomography performed elsewhere revealed that both internal auditory canals were normal.

A Polytomograph showing well-delineated left internal auditory canal (*arrows*), which appears entirely normal when compared with the right.

B CT scan with wide window setting reveals widening of the left internal auditory canal when compared with the normal right side.

C Contrast scan shows markedly enhanced, well circumscribed tumor (*arrows*) in the left cerebellopontine angle. The fourth ventricle is displaced to the right side.

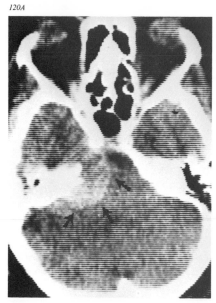

120A

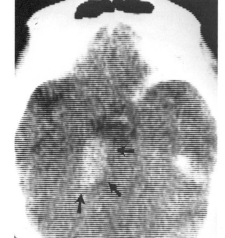

120B

Fig. 120. Tentorial meningioma extending to the cerebellopontine angle in a 75-year-old female with a 6-month history of right facial numbness, progressively decreased hearing on the right side, and ataxic gait. Postcontrast scans show:

A an enhanced tumor with well-defined convex medial border (*arrows*) in the cerebellopontine angle and,

B the tumor extends upward through the tentorial notch, resulting in a flattened lateral edge caused by the tentorium and medial convex border (*arrows*).

Tumors less than 15 mm in diameter are generally missed by intravenous enhanced CT. Metrizamide (Amipaque) CT cisternography, air CT cisternography, or Pantopaque cisternography should be performed on the patient in whom a small cerebellopontine angle tumor or intracanalicular tumor is suspected but could not be demonstrated by conventional intravenous CT. It is advised that concerned areas must be viewed with different window settings, preferably on the display console, so that the viewer can manipulate the window width and window level for the proper setting.

Arachnoid cyst is an abnormal collection of cerebrospinal fluid, which may occur over the cerebral hemispheres, beneath the temporal lobes, or in the posterior fossa. Depending largely on its location, it may be associated with chronic headache or epilepsy, or it may remain asymptomatic.

Its CT appearances are often pathognomonic. It is a well-defined, nonenhanced lesion that may have a sharply defined inner border, representing the attachment of the cyst to arachnoid membrane (fig. 122).

Hydrocephalus frequently accompanies a posterior fossa arachnoid cyst, as seen in our case. Its treatment consists of suboccipital craniotomy and excision; however, mild residual symptoms may persist, since the central nervous tissue has been compressed for a long time, in most cases.

Fig. 121. Glomus jugulare tumor with extensive bony erosion around the foramen jugulare and enhanced tumor in the cerebellopontine region in a 52-year-old female. This patient had a 3-year history of progressive hearing impairment in her right ear, "funny" or sweet taste, hoarseness, and choking sensation. A small glomus jugular tumor was removed from her right middle ear 3 years ago, at another hospital.

A Enhanced tumor (*arrows*) in the cerebellopontine angle but separated from the petrous bone.

B CT scan in coronal position reveals gross bony destruction around the jugular foramen (*double arrows*) compared with the opposite normal one (*single arrow*).

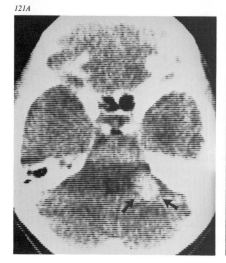

121A

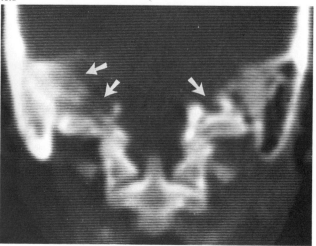

121B

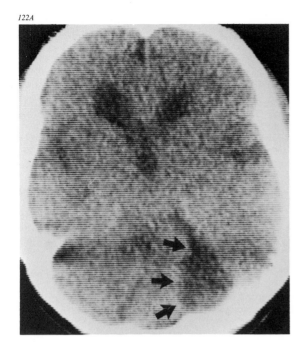

122A

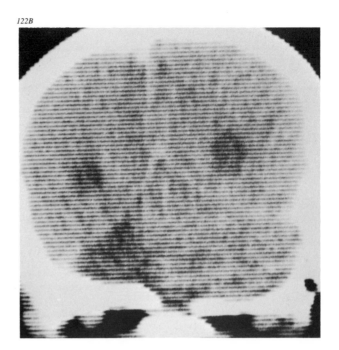

122B

Fig. 122. Extra-axial arachnoid cyst in 35-year-old male with a history of severe frontal headaches for many years.

A Contrast scan shows large, nonenhanced cyst occupies a large part of the left half of posterior fossa. The lateral straight border of the cyst demarcates the tentorial edge. Notice the sharply defined inner border (*arrows*) representing the attachment of the cyst with the arachnoid membrane and the underlying cerebellar hemisphere. Marked degree of hydrocephalus is visible on higher section (not shown).

B Contrast scan in coronal position shows the relationship between tentorium and cyst. Thickening of the occipital bone behind and below the cyst can be appreciated in both *A* and *D*. At surgery, the left cerebellar hemisphere was found to be displaced from left to right. A large arachnoid cyst was removed, which contained about 40 ml of clear cerebrospinal fluid. The cyst extended from the tentorium to the cerebellopontine angle.

Bibliography

Adair LB, Ropper AH, Davis KR: Cerebellar hemangioblastoma: computed tomographic, angiographic and clinical correlation in seven cases. CT 2:281, 1978.

Baker H, Houser W: Computed tomography in the diagnosis of posterior fossa lesions. Radiol Clin N Am 14:129, 1976.

Banna M: Arachnoid cysts on computed tomography. AJR 127:979, 1976.

Berger P, Kriks DR, Gilday DL: Computed tomography in infants and children: intracranial neoplasms. AJR 127:129, 1976.

Bilaniuk LT, Zimmerman RA, Littman P, et al: Computed tomography of brainstem gliomas in children. Radiology 134:89, 1980.

Cornell SH, Chiu LC, Christie MH: Diagnosis of extracerebral fluid collections by computed tomography. AJR 131:107, 1978.

Davis KR, Parker SW, New PFJ, et al: Computed tomography of acoustic neuroma. Radiology 124:81 1977.

Delavelle J, Megret M: CT sagittal reconstruction of posterior fossa tumors. Neuroradiology 19:81, 1980.

Drayer BP, Rosenbaum AE, Maroon J, et al: Posterior fossa extra-axial cyst: diagnosis with metrizamide CT cisternography. AJR 128:431, 1977.

Dubois PJ, Drayer BP, Bank WO, et al: An evaluation of current diagnostic radiologic modalities in the investigation of acoustic neurilemmomas. Radiology 126:173, 1978.

Gado M, Huete I, Mikhael M: Computerized tomography of infratentorial tumors. Semin Roentgenol 12:109, 1977.

Glenn WV Jr, Johnson RJ, Morton PE, et al: Further investigation and initial clinical use of an advanced CT display capability. Invest Radiol 10:479, 1975.

Gyldensted C, Lester J, Thomsen J: Computer tomography in the diagnosis of cerebellopontine angle tumors. Neuroradiology 11:191, 1976.

Hammerschlag SB, Wolpert SM, Carter BL: Computed coronal tomography. Radiology 120:219, 1978.

Kazner E, Aulich A, Grumme T: Results of computerized axial tomography with infratentorial tumors. In: Cranial Computerized Tomography. Edited by Lanksch W, Kazner E. Springer, Berlin, 1976, pp. 90–103.

Kingsley DPE, Kendall BE: The CT scanner in posterior fossa tumours of childhood. Br J Radiol 52:769, 1979.

Kricheff II, Pinto RS, Bergeron RT, et al: Air-CT cisternography and canalography for small acoustic neuromas. AJNR 1:57, 1980.

Maravilla KR: Computer reconstructed sagittal and coronal computed tomography head scans: clinical applications. J Comput Assist Tomogr 2:189, 1978.

Miller EM, Newton TH: Extra-axial posterior fossa lesions simulating intra-axial lesions on computed tomography. Radiology 127:676, 1978.

Möller A, Hatam A, Olivecrona H: Diagnosis of acoustic neuroma with computed tomography. Neuroradiology 17:25, 1978.

Möller A, Hatam A, Olivecrona H: The differential diagnosis of pontine angle meningioma and acoustic neuroma with computed tomography. Neuroradiology 17:21, 1978.

Naidich TP, Leeds NE, Kricheff II, et al: The tentorium in axial section I. Normal CT appearance and non-neoplastic pathology. Radiology 123:631, 1977.

Naidich TP, Leeds NE, Kricheff II, et al: The tentorium in axial section II, Lesion Localization. Radiology 123:639, 1977.

Naidich TP, Lin JP, Leeds NE, et al: Computed tomography in the diagnosis of extra-axial posterior fossa masses. Radiology 120:33, 1976.

Naidich TP, Lin JP, Leeds NE, et al: Primary tumors and other masses of the cerebellum and fourth ventricle: differential diagnosis by computed tomography. Neuroradiology 14:153, 1977.

New PFJ, Scott WR, Schnur JA, et al: Computerized axial tomography with the EMI scanner. Radiology 110:109, 1974.

New PFJ, Scott WR, Schnur JA, et al: Computed tomography with the EMI scanner in the diagnosis of primary and metastatic intracranial neoplasms. Radiology 114:75, 1975.

Paxton R, Ambrose J: The EMI scanner, a brief review of the first 650 patients. Br J Radiol 47:530, 1974.

Probst FP, Liliequist B: Assessment of posterior fossa tumors in infants and children by means of computed tomography. Neuroradiology 18:9, 1979.

Rao KG, Woodlief RM: CT simulation of cerebellopontine tumor by tortuous vertebrobasilar artery. AJR 132:672, 1979.

Robbins B, Marshall WH Jr: Computed tomography of acoustic neurinoma. Radiology 128:367, 1978.

Salvolini U, Menichelli F, Pasquini U: Cerebellopontine expansive lesions. In: Clinical Computer Tomography—Head and Trunk. Edited by Baert A, Jeanmart L, Wackenheim A. Springer, Berlin, 1978, pp 79–103.

Schulz RA, Joseph PM, Hilal SK: Frontal and lateral views of the brain reconstructed from EMI axial slices. Radiology 125:701, 1977.

Staelens B, Palmers Y, Baert A, et al: Tumoral masses of the posterior fossa. In: Clinical Computer Tomography—Head and Trunk. Edited by Baert A, Jeanmart L, Wackenheim A. Springer, Berlin, 1978, pp 65–70.

Tadmor R, Harwood-Nash DCF, Savoiardo M, et al: Brain tumors in the first two years of life: CT diagnosis. AJNR 1:411, 1980.

Wilson JL, Moseley IF: A diagnostic approach to cerebellar lesions. European seminar on computerized axial tomography in clinical practice. Edited by du Boulay GH, Moseley IF. Springer, Berlin, 1977, pp 123–133.

Wolf BS, Nakagawa H, Staulcup PH: Feasibility of coronal views in computed scanning of the head. Radiology 120:217, 1976.

Zimmerman RA, Bilaniuk LT, Bruno L, et al: Computed tomography of cerebellar astrocytoma. AJR 130:929, 1978.

Chapter IX

Dandy-Walker Syndrome

Dandy-Walker syndrome (Dandy-Walker cyst or atresia of the foramina of Luschka and Magendie) is a congenital cystic dilatation of the fourth ventricle, associated with the absence of the inferior vermis, cerebellar dysplasia, and frequently with anomalies of other parts of the brain. Agenesis of the corpus callosum is an associated finding in about one-half of the cases. The fourth ventricle is grossly dilated and prevents downward movement of the tentorium cerebelli and lateral sinuses, which normally occurs in the late stages of fetal life. The skull radiograph reveals an enlarged posterior fossa, with posterior bulging and thinning of the occipital squamosa. The grooves for the lateral sinuses and sinus confluens are elevated.

The CT findings are quite characteristic. (fig. 123). There is no normal fourth ventricle; instead, there is a large posterior fossa cyst. The caudal vermis is absent; the cerebellum is small, dysplastic, and asymmetric; and the tentorium is either displaced upward or does not descend, resulting in a "inverted-V sign."

A posterior fossa arachnoid cyst may mimic a Dandy-Walker cyst, but an arachnoid cyst is not associated with dysplastic cerebellum.

Aqueductus Stenosis

The most common cause of internal hydrocephalus in the

newborn and in young infants is congenital stenosis of the aqueduct of Sylvius. Obstruction, may be caused by the presence of a membrane in the aqueduct, actual stenosis, or, more commonly forking of the aqueduct into two or more abnormal channels. The total cross-sectional diameter of these channels is smaller than normal, and many end blindly.

The aqueduct stenosis results in dilatation of the lateral and third ventricles (often massive), but not of the fourth ventricle. The suprapineal recess may expand to a huge cystic structure. These findings are readily demonstrable by CT (fig. 124). In pronounced hydrocephalus, occasionally the walls of the lateral ventricles and of the third ventricle appear to be scalloped. This appearance is attributed to the difference in the rate of stretching between the less elastic

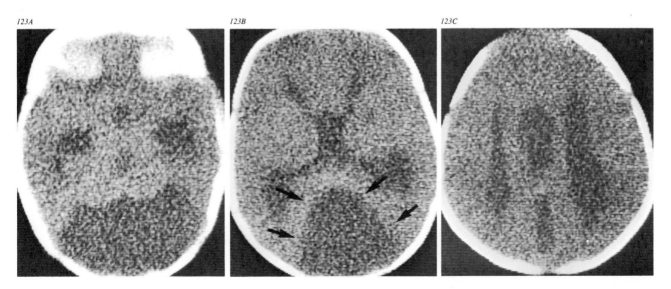

123A *123B* *123C*

Fig. 123. A case of Dandy-Walker cyst associated with agenesis of the corpus callosum.

A Note the huge posterior fossa cyst with a small, dysplastic, asymmetric cerebellum.

B The cyst herniates upwards, elevating the tentorium and displacing the dilated area and occipital horns. Notice the inverted-V sign (arrows).

C Agenesis of the corpus callosum with high position of the third ventricle, and wide separation of the lateral ventricles.

124A

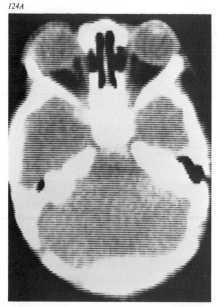

124B

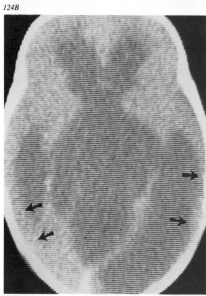

124C

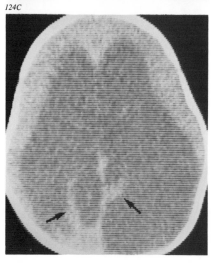

arteries and the expansible subependymal layers of the ventricular walls. Intraventricular septations are easily demonstrable by CT and may be responsible for some of the shunt failure.

CT is extremely valuable for monitoring post-shunt complications, which include collapse of the ventricles due to an overly rapid removal of cerebrospinal fluid. Also, subdural hematoma may develop and cause compression of the ventricular system. Or, the post-shunt patient may become shunt dependent, with subnormal ventricular size (slit-like ventricles). Finally, shunt malfunction may develop with a progressive increase in ventricular size.

Hydrocephalus due to aqueduct stenosis must be differentiated from communicating hydrocephalus (fig. 125), which usually results from an obstruction in the subarachnoid space distal to the fourth ventricle, either within the basal cisterns, at the tentorial notch, or over the convolutional sulci of the brain. Adhesions may result from infection or hemorrhage. Perinatal intracranial hemorrhage due to either traumatic delivery or related to hypoxia at birth is a common cause of congenital hydrocephalus. Newborn infants, especially prematures with respiratory distress syndrome, are particularly susceptible to subependymal germinal matrix hemorrhage.

Porencephaly

Porencephaly or porencephalic cyst refers to an ependymally lined, CSF-containing cavity in the brain substance, which communicates either with the ventricles, the subarachnoid spaces, or both. According to various authors, the etiologic factors in the formation of porencephaly are trauma, cerebral vascular occlusion, postinflammatory changes, focal atrophy, hemorrhage, repeated episodes of localized arterial spasm, and postsurgical changes (*Ramsey*

Fig. 124. A case of aqueduct stenosis in a 3-month-old girl with enlarging head size of 1 month duration. The anterior fontanelle was tense.

A Scan of the posterior fossa reveals no enlarged fourth ventricle or other cystic structure.

B Massive dilatation of the occipital horns and third ventricle with its suprapineal recess, which has scalloped borders. In spite of huge occipital horns, a thin layer of cortex is still visible (*arrows*), in contradistinction to hydranencephaly. There is also disproportionate dilatation of the atria and occipital horns with respect to the frontal horns, a common finding in patients with hydrocephalus of various etiologies.

C Scan at higher level showing septations (*arrows*) in the lateral ventricles.

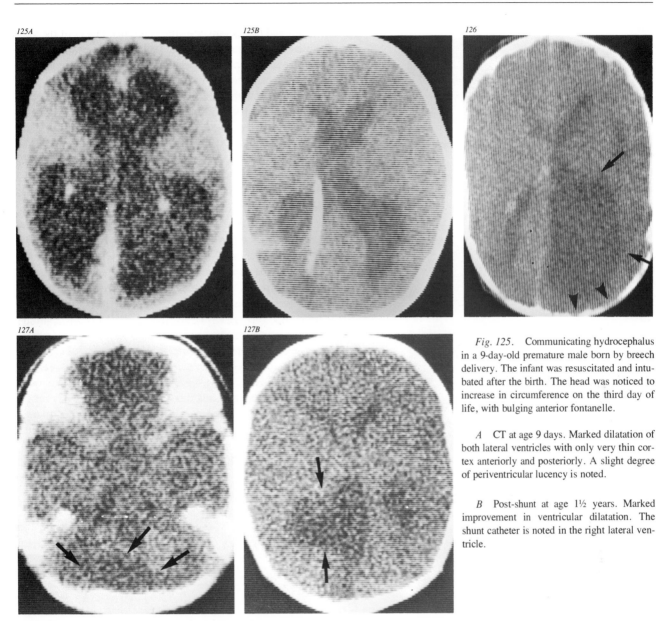

Fig. 125. Communicating hydrocephalus in a 9-day-old premature male born by breech delivery. The infant was resuscitated and intubated after the birth. The head was noticed to increase in circumference on the third day of life, with bulging anterior fontanelle.

A CT at age 9 days. Marked dilatation of both lateral ventricles with only very thin cortex anteriorly and posteriorly. A slight degree of periventricular lucency is noted.

B Post-shunt at age 1½ years. Marked improvement in ventricular dilatation. The shunt catheter is noted in the right lateral ventricle.

Fig. 126. Porencephaly, left occipital region (*arrows*) with localized thinning of the cranial vault (*arrowheads*). The left frontal horn is slightly dilated and there is a ventricular shift to the right side throughout the remaining images. This newborn girl was noted to have a large head and multiple anomalies. There is severe spinal dysraphism extending from T10 to the sacrum, severe gibbus kyphotic deformity of the lumbar spine, and congenital dislocation of the right hip.

Fig. 127. Porencephaly secondary to birth trauma in a 6-day-old girl who was noted to have seizures 3 hours after a difficult birth. Examination reveals severe, generalized hypotonia. Porencephalic cysts (*arrows*) are noted in the:

A posterior fossa and

B in the right occipital lobe.

and Huckman, 1977). The bony changes seen in skull radiographs are variable: there may be localized thinning or thickening of the skull tables (fig. 126). Midline structures may show no shift, or they may shift either towards or away from the cyst. CT readily demonstrates cysts that have absorption values the same as that of cerebrospinal fluid (fig. 127), but is of somewhat limited value in precisely determining the presence or absence of membrane between the cyst and the ventricle. Sometimes the cyst appears to communicate with the ventricle on CT when, in fact, it may be separated from it by a thin membrane.

Cerebral Hemiatrophy (DDM: Dyke, Davidoff, Masson Syndrome)

Dyke, Davidoff and Masson (1938) described the characteristic radiologic findings of cerebral hemiatrophy with

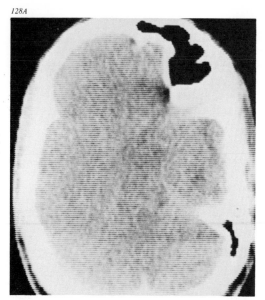

128A

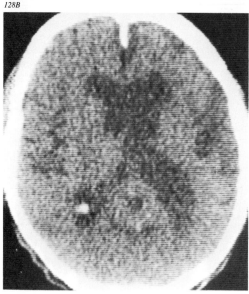

128B

homolateral hypertrophy of the skull and sinuses. Since the impaired hemisphere grows at a slower rate, very little pressure is exerted on the adjacent skull. Consequently, the ipsilateral side of the head is smaller than the opposite side, and the bone is thicker. In an effort to further compensate for the diminished volume of the brain, the petrous ridges become elevated, the sphenoid wings prominent, and the paranasal sinuses on the involved side increase in volume. Within the involved hemicerebrum, the lateral ventricle becomes dilated and shifts ipsilaterally (*Dyke et al., 1933*).

The lesions usually occur early in life, and not infrequently follow birth trauma or an acute infectious episode. Clinical presentations may vary. The hemiplegia and convulsions may manifest at birth or at intervals of months after the trauma. Almost all patients dated their illness back either to birth or to within the first 15 months of life, with rare exceptions. This fact explains the compensatory changes in the skull.

The CT appearance in a fully developed case is pathognomonic, and reflects the changes seen on plain skull radiography and pneumoencephalography (fig. 128). The findings are ipsilateral ventricular dilatation with a decrease in cerebral volume on the involved side. The ventricular system is shifted towards the side of the lesion. The cortical markings overlying the involved hemicerebrum are dilated. The ethmoid, frontal maxillary, and mastoid air cells on the involved side are overpneumatized. There is ipsilateral calvarial thickening, and the middle cranial fossa is smaller on the involved side. True elevation of the petrous and sphenoid bones should not be confused with rotation of the head due to positioning. Flattening of the calvarial curvature becomes more obvious when the scan section reaches the vertex.

128C

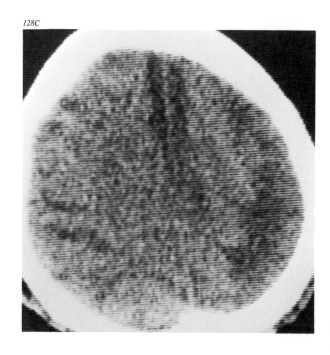

Fig. 128. Cerebral hemiatrophy in a 60-year-old man with mental retardation, history of epilepsy, and congenital right hemiparesis.

A Enlarged left frontal sinus, elevation and thickening of the left sphenoid wing.

B Decreased left hemicranium with flattening of the calvarial curvature anteriorly, ipsilateral ventricular shift toward the lesion, ipsilateral dilatation of the lateral ventricle and the Sylvian fissure.

C Ipsilateral widening of the convolutional sulci and flattening of the calvarial curvature.

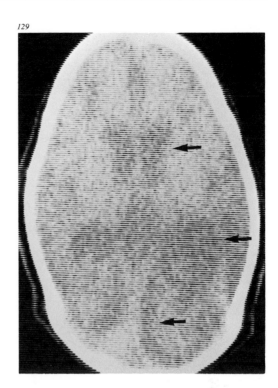

Fig. 129. Microcephaly in a 4-month-old girl with history of seizures and retardation since birth. Skull radiographs reveal synostosis of all sutures. There is dilatation of both lateral ventricles, the third ventricle, the interhemispheric fissure, and the subarachnoid spaces around the hemispheres. The changes are slightly more pronounced on the left side (*arrows*).

The CT findings of the brain, ventricles, and subarachnoid space in congenital hemiatrophy may be seen as the end stage of massive cerebral infarction; calvarial changes, however, are not present in the latter.

Microcephaly

Microcephaly, or small brain, refers to cerebral hypoplasia, an undergrowth of the brain. Because the brain ceases to grow, there is thus a lack of stimulus for the skull to expand. The condition may be familial, or it may be associated with various factors, including trauma, diseases such as toxoplasmosis, or cytomegalic inclusion disease, viral infections, and fetal irradiation in utero (for radiotherapy of the maternal pelvis).

CT reveals that the ventricular system is dilated, usually symmetrically (fig. 129). One part of the ventricle may be larger than its counterpart, usually only to a slight degree. The basilar cisterns and the convolutional sulci are widened. On bone window setting, the sutures are thin, narrow, or closed.

Hydranencephaly

In hydranencephaly the cerebral hemispheres fail to develop owing to prenatal hypoplasia or occlusion of the internal carotid arteries. The areas affected are mainly those supplied by the internal carotid circulation. The structures receiving supply from the vertebrobasilar system remain relatively preserved. These include the cerebellum, midbrain, brain stem, basal ganglia, and varying portions of the occipital and temporal lobes. The CT features are characteristic (fig. 130): the cerebral hemispheres are replaced by a large fluid-filled meningeal sac without ependymal lining. Brain tissue density and the fourth ventricle in the posterior fossa are usually preserved. Egg-shaped or rounded bodies, representing the basal ganglia, thalami, and remaining brain tissue, are seen in the base of the brain. Remnants of subfrontal cortex may be present. The falx is intact in hydranencephaly, as opposed to alobar holoprosencephaly. Hydranencephaly is a term derived from a combination of two words: *hydrocephalus* and *anencephaly*. The word anencephaly is not quite appropriate and the term hydrencephaly has been suggested.

Hydranencephaly must be differentiated from massive subdural effusion, hydrocephalus, and alobar holoprosencephaly. In severe hydrocephalus there is always some cortical mantle, which is absent in classic cases of hydranencephaly. A thalamic nubbin or thalamic nodule appearance is an important differential point from massive congenital subdural hematomas. Generally, infants with hydranencephaly have a normal facial appearance as opposed to alobar holoprosencephaly, which always presents with midline cleft deformities and hypotelorism.

130A

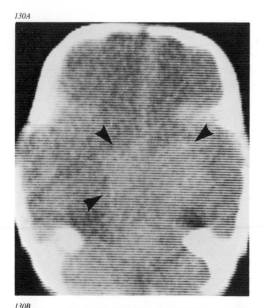

130B

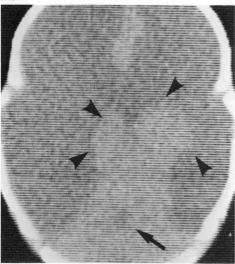

130C

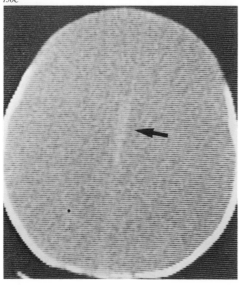

Fig. 130. Hydranencephaly in a 5-week-old infant. This male baby was born to a 21-year-old unmarried woman who had tried to "get rid of the baby" in her first 2 months of pregnancy, taking pills and iodine douches. Congenital hydrocephalus was diagnosed in utero by ultrasound. The baby was born by normal vaginal delivery but the head was growing by ¼ to ½ cm daily. The anterior fontanelle was moderately bulging but soft to touch. The infant also developed spastic quadriplegia and there was no visual pursuit.

The characteristic CT features of hydranencephaly are presented here in three selected scans.

A and B These scans demonstrate normal brain density of the posterior fossa structures. The fourth ventricle (*arrow*) is well seen and appears normal. The egg-shaped nubbin of tissue is seen in the base of the brain (*arrowheads*), apparently representing diencephalic remnants (thalamic and hypothalamic). Between the CSF-filled sac and the frontal and temporal bony calvarium, there is no visible cortical thickness. This is in contradistinction to hydrocephalus (e.g., aqueduct stenosis), where one still can see some peripheral cortical tissue. In the frontal area, a small wedge of remnant tissue is visible.

C Higher scan shows total absence of normal telencephalic structures with a relatively intact falx cerebri (*arrow*).

Bibliography

Allen JH, Martin JT, McLain LW: Computed tomography in cerebellar atrophic processes. Radiology 130:379, 1979.

Byrd SE, Harwood-Nash DC, Fitz CF, et al: CT evaluation of holoprosencephaly in infants and children. J Comput Assist Tomogr 1:456, 1977.

Di Chiro G, Arimitsu T, Brooks RA, et al: Computed tomography profiled of periventricular hypodensity in hydrocephalus and leukoencephalopathy. Radiology 130:661, 1979.

Di Chiro G, Arimitsu T, Pollock JM, et al: Periventricular leukomalacia related to neonatal anoxia: Recognition by computed tomography. J Comput Assist Tomogr 2:352, 1978.

Di Chiro G, Elben RM, Manz HJ, et al: New CT pattern in adrenoleukodystrophy. Radiology 137:687, 1980.

Dublin AB, French BN: Diagnostic image evaluation of hydranencephaly and pictorially similar entities, with emphasis on computed tomography. Radiology 137:81, 1980.

Dyke CG, Davidoff LM, Masson CB: Cerebral hemiatrophy with homolateral hypertrophy of the skull and sinuses. Surg Gynecol Obstet 57:588, 1933.

Fitz CR, Harwood-Nash DC: Computed tomography in hydrocephalus. CT: 2:91, 1978.

Flodmark O, Becker LE, Harwood-Nash, DC, et al: Correlation between computed tomography and autopsy in premature and full-term neonates that have suffered perinatal asphyxia. Radiology 137:93, 1980.

Fowler FD, Alexander Jr E: Atresia of the foramina of Luschka and Magendi. Am J Dis Child 92:131, 1956.

Harwood-Nash DC: Congenital craniocerebral abnormalities and computed tomography. Semin Roentgenol 12:39, 1977.

Heinz ER, Drayer BP, Haenggeli CA, et al: Computed tomography in white-matter disease. Radiology 130:371, 1979.

Huckman MS, Fox JH, Ramsey RG: Computed tomography in the diagnosis of degenerative disease of the brain. Semin Roentgenol 12:63, 1977.

Huckman MS, Fox JS, Ramsey RG, et al: Computed tomography in the diagnosis of pseudotumor cerebri. Radiology 119:593, 1976.

Jacoby CG, Go RT, Hahn FJ: Computed tomography in cerebral hemiatrophy. AJR 129:5, 1977.

Lane B, Carroll BA, Pedley TA: Computerized cranial tomography in cerebral diseases of white matter. Neurology 28:534, 1978.

Naidich TH, Epstein F, Lin JP, et al: Evaluation of pediatric hydrocephalus by computed tomography. Radiology 119:337, 1976.

Nixon GW, Johns Jr RE, Myers GG: Congenital porencephaly. Pediatrics 54:43, 1974.

Palmieri A, Menichelli F, Pasquini U, et al: Role of CT in the postoperative evaluation of infantile hydrocephalus. Neuroradiology 14:257, 1978.

Ramsey RG, Huckman MS: Computed tomography of porencephaly and other cerebrospinal fluid-containing lesions. Radiology 123:73, 1977.

Roberts MA, Caird FL, Grossart KW, et al: Computerized tomography in the diagnosis of cerebral atrophy. J Neurol Neurosurg Psychiatry 39:909, 1976.

Schellinger D, McCullough DC, Pederson RT: Computed tomography in the hydrocephalic patient after shunting. Radiology 137:693, 1980.

Taboada D, Alonso A, Olague R, et al: Radiological diagnosis of periventricular and subcortical leukomalacia. Neuroradiology 20:33, 1980.

Chapter X

Brain Abscess

CT has contributed significantly to the diagnosis and management of brain abscess. Before the CT era, mortality from brain abscess had been 30 to 60 percent. Despite improved neurosurgical techniques and modern antibiotic therapy, mortality remained high during the last 20 years. However, since CT was introduced, the death rate due to brain abscess has dramatically decreased to nearly 5 percent. The reason for the decrease is CT not only provides early diagnosis of brain abscess, but also accurately deter-

mines its location and size, as well as the presence of multiple abscesses. Being a noninvasive procedure, CT is useful for monitoring the course of the abscess at the early stage of its development, to guide the surgeon for the optimal time for surgery, and to follow the size of the cavity after the operation.

The CT appearance of an abscess is characteristic (fig. 131). On the precontrast scan, one sees a considerable amount of edema. Occasionally, one may perceive a faint rim of high density within the edema. After contrast administration, nearly all patients demonstrate rim enhancement, which outlines the capsule of the abscess, thus permitting an accurate assessment of the size and location of the abscess. The degree of the enhancement varies with the age of the abscess and probably is most intense at 2 to 3 weeks after the initial symptoms. During the early stage, when the abscess wall is being formed, the enhancement may be only faint or not even discernible. It has been shown that with as little as a 2-day interval, a repeat CT demonstrates enhanced capsule not visible 2 days earlier. It is important to remember that contrast administration is absolutely necessary to enhance the abscess capsule. CT without contrast injection in patients with signs of infection is, therefore, an incom-

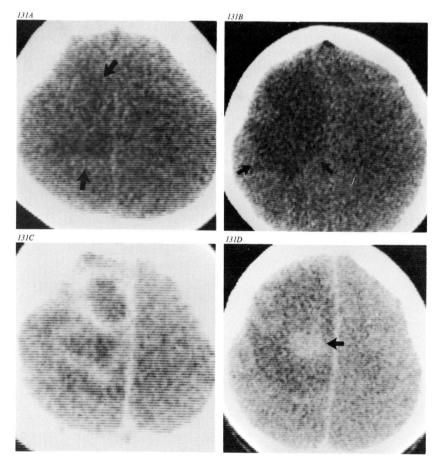

Fig. 131. Brain abscesses with enhanced capsules. This 33-year-old woman was admitted with dense left hemiplegia that developed over the last week. Her illness was preceded 2 weeks ago by sneezing, cough, headache, running nose, and fever. One week ago she noted weakness of the left arm and leg, which evidently resolved completely within a day, but began to recur and progressed to a complete left hemiplegia on the day of admission. Examination revealed a flaccid left hemiplegia with left Babinski.

A and B Precontrast scans reveal low attenuation lesion in the right frontoparietal region (*arrows*). No dense rim is visible on noncontrast scans.

C and D Postcontrast scans reveal two adjacent abscesses with enhanced capsules and surrounding edema. The lower scan (*D*) apparently traverses through the inferior wall of the abscess, and therefore appears homogeneous in density (*arrow*). At surgery, about 20 ml of greenish-yellow foul-smelling pus was aspirated. Culture yielded *Streptococcus viridans*.

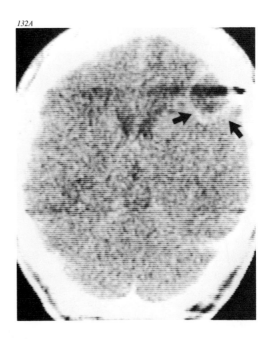

132A

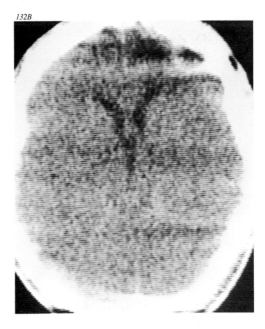

132B

Fig. 132. This 29-year-old man had left frontal craniotomy for removal of necrotic brain, bullet fragments, and evacuation of an epidural hematoma 3 weeks ago.

A Postcontrast CT 3 weeks post craniotomy: ring-enhanced lesion in the left frontal region (*arrows*) with slight ventricular shift to the left. Horizontal lucent artifacts were produced by bony defect (*arrowhead*) following craniotomy. The patient had low-grade fever for almost 1 week, but the lumbar puncture was normal. While abscess formation cannot be excluded on CT, it was felt that lack of edema around the ring-enhanced lesion and the patient's clinical condition do not suggest abscess formation. It was felt that the ring-enhanced lesion most probably represented postoperative changes. The patient's condition was therefore monitored clinically and by follow-up CT scans.

B Repeat CT scan with contrast 17 days after the first CT revealed almost complete resolution of the ring-enhanced lesion. This case illustrates the occasional difficulties in differentiating ring-enhanced lesions, and the value of sequential CT scans.

plete study that may lead to a false sense of security, actually missing the abscess.

An abscess must be differentiated from other ring-enhanced lesions, such as primary and secondary malignant neoplasm, resolving hematoma, postoperative changes (fig. 132), and infarction. For example, in glioblastoma multiforme, the enhanced ring is more irregular in shape and thickness than the abscess, and is frequently associated with inner nodularity. In contrast, while nodular enhancement may be observed near the periphery of the ring in an abscess, inner nodularity projecting into the central low-density zone is unlikely. In about half of the cases, either multiple abscesses, or multilocular abscesses with daughter loculi are observed. In metastatic lesions, multiple, ring-enhanced foci are usually distinctly separate, while the walls of the daughter loculi seem to blend with each other. In cases where differential diagnosis may be difficult, angiography should be performed, since in most studies, the tumor stain seen in glioblastoma multiforme and metastases, would allow a differential diagnosis between abscess and tumor.

It is known that steroid therapy may decrease the enhancement in abscess or malignant neoplasm. One must, therefore, be cautious in interpreting the decrease of enhancement as a sign that the abscess resolved during steroid therapy. The mass effect must be taken into consideration in evaluating the progress of the disease.

Subdural and Epidural Empyema

The most common cause of subdural empyema is an otorhinologic or paranasal sinus infection. Other causes include penetrating wounds of the skull, cranial osteomyelitis, infection of a subdural hematoma, meningitis, and septicemia. In subdural empyema, the CT scan demonstrates a crescent-shaped area of low attenuation adjacent to the cortex. Unlike the epidural empyema, the subdural empyema often extends over a diffuse area, because the subdural space does not restrict the spread of subdural exudate. Subdural empyema may spread into the parafalcian area. This possibility should be carefully sought during scan interpretation. Characteristically, the postcontrast scan reveals enhancement of the subdural membrane. A chronic type of

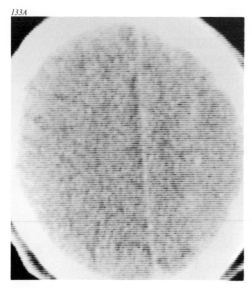

133A

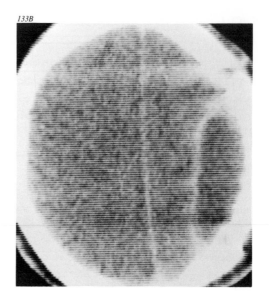

133B

Fig. 133. Subdural empyema, postsurgical, in a 58-year-old man who had been found unconscious following an acute onset of slurred speech. There was history of dysarthria and right upper extremity weakness of 3 days duration.

A Postcontrast scan reveals an almost isodense subdural hematoma in the left parietal region. Note the effacement of the sulci on the left side. A left frontotemporo-parietal trephination was performed, and a chronic subdural hematoma was evacuated. The patient was readmitted about 1 month later with recent intensification of preexisting dysarthria and right hemiparesis.

B Repeat scan with contrast revealed subdural collections with densely enhanced capsule. At surgery, a large subdural empyema was evacuated.

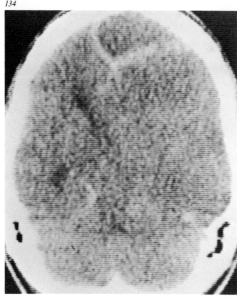

134

Fig. 134. Frontal epidural empyema in a 37-year-old male drug addict with a history of endocarditis. He had presented to the emergency room initially in a lethargic state. Over the next 12 hours, his mental status deteriorated and he became comatose, responsive only to deep pain. The patient had fever for 1 week prior to admission, with progressively severe headache. A lumbar puncture yielded seven polymorphonuclear cells per cubic millimeter. CT was obtained on the day of admission. Precontrast scan (not shown) revealed large low density lesion in the front area with marked ventricular shift to the right. Postcontrast scan revealed epidural empyema with densely enhanced capsule, which crossed the midline. A small subdural collection with faint enhancement of membrane was also noted in the left parietotemporal region. Plain film of the skull revealed a large bony defect, and 50 ml of pus was withdrawn via a tap through the bony defect. Through a left parietal burrhole clear xanthochromic fluid was recovered. At craniotomy, cheesy, purulent exudate was found filling the frontal sinuses. Despite vigorous antibiotic therapy, the patient died 2 weeks after admission.

empyema tends to demonstrate a thicker capsule (fig. 133). However, membrane enhancement may also be seen in chronic subdural hematoma, and the differential diagnosis from the latter may be difficult without an appropriate history. Membrane enhancement is usually not seen in subdural effusion or hygroma.

Subdural empyema is a fulminating disease and must be considered a surgical emergency. Like subdural hematoma, it may also be isodense with the brain. It is important to recognize this limitation, and in suspected cases high-dose contrast CT or delayed scan may be useful. Occasionally, angiography is necessary for a definitive diagnosis.

Epidural empyema usually is the result of direct extension from osteomyelitis of the skull secondary to sinusitis, mastoiditis, or trauma. It tends to be localized, since the

dura is difficult to strip away from the periosteum of the inner table (fig. 134). If the empyema crosses the midline, the diagnosis of epidural location is virtually certain, since the subdural empyema would normally be stopped in the midline by the falx.

Herpes Simplex Encephalitis

Herpes simplex encephalitis, an acute fulminant necrotizing and hemorrhagic encephalitis, is caused by herpes simplex virus (herpesvirus hominis), a virus first isolated from the brain of a dying child in 1941. The disease is the most frequent fatal form of nonepidemic encephalitis. Death usually occurs in the second or third week, and those few who survive are severely handicapped by neurologic deficits. The diagnosis can be established by brain biopsy, which may yield positive virus cultures and/or demonstrate intranuclear inclusion bodies on histologic study. Early diagnosis may be life-saving, since recent studies have indicated a favorable therapeutic response with prompt use of specific antiviral agents, such as adenine arabinoside (ARA-A).

The disease has a predilection for the temporal lobes and the insular, as well as the orbital surface of the frontal lobe, either unilateral or bilateral.

CT findings consist of a low density lesion located in the temporal frontotemporal region, or insular cortex. The mass effect may be present. The appearance of contrast enhancement is variable. The enhanced areas present as ring or gyral configurations, between 7 and 24 days after the ictus (fig. 135 and 136).

Clinically, patients develop symptoms suggestive of an infectious process, followed by focal neurologic findings, including seizures and increased intracranial pressure. In the majority of cases there is mental confusion and disorientation. In no patient is the cerebrospinal fluid entirely normal; protein concentrations are elevated with pleocytosis in the majority of cases, and the red cell count is greater than 10 in most patients.

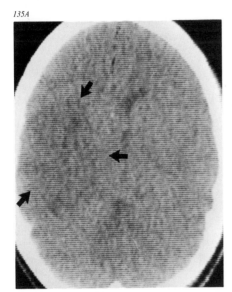
135A

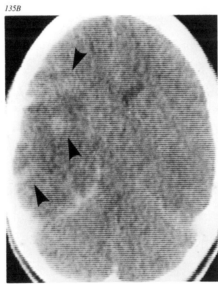
135B

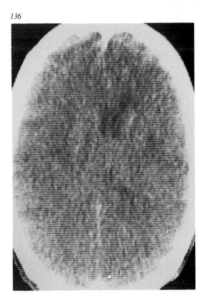
136

Fig. 135. Herpes simplex encephalitis in a 23-year-old black woman, 8 weeks postpartum. She had presented with acute onset of altered mental status and fever of 102.6° F following an urinary infection 1 week ago. Her temperature was 102.6° F and her white blood count was 15,400. Her neck was supple, but a lumbar puncture yielded 240 WBC with lymphocytic pleocytosis (188 lymphocytes, 52 polymorphonuclear cells), protein 59 mg percent, and glucose 270 mg percent.

A Precontrast scan reveals low density lesion in the right frontal temporal region (*arrows*) displacing the third ventricle to the left side. The right frontal horn is compressed.

B Postcontrast scan shows gyral and nodular enhancement (*arrowheads*) scattered throughout the low density lesion. The serum specimens, taken on admission and on subsequent days, revealed a fourfold rise of herpesvirus hominis antibody titers. There was also the appearance of herpesvirus hominis antibodies in the cerebrospinal fluid. These findings suggested the diagnosis of herpes simplex encephalitis. The patient was treated with adenine arabinoside before the results of antibody titers and the cerebrospinal fluid findings of herpes antibodies were known, and she made a good recovery.

Fig. 136. Herpes simplex encephalitis proved by biopsy in a 46-year-old missionary who had developed right ear pain followed by a generalized headache 3 weeks ago. There was an increase in the number of "seizures" the patient had experienced for the past 26 years following a car accident. There were 11 leukocytes, all polymorphonuclear cells. CT scan following contrast medium revealed a mass lesion in the right frontotemporal region, causing marked contralateral ventricular shift. The right frontal horn and the occipital horn were compressed. A right carotid arteriogram confirmed a large avascular right frontotemporal mass. A right temporal lobe biopsy was performed, and the patient was started immediately postoperatively on adenine arabinoside. The tissue cultures from the brain grew out Herpes simplex type 1 within 24 hours. Electron microscopic examination of the brain tissue revealed intranuclear and intracytoplasmic virions, consistent with herpetic encephalitis. The patient continued to improve with ability to ambulate by the third hospital week. He remained confused at night and frequently inappropriate in his behavior. He was discharged to be followed by his local physician.

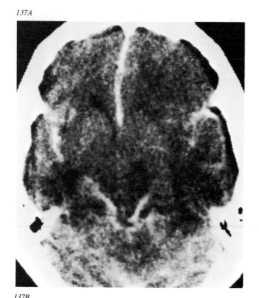

137A

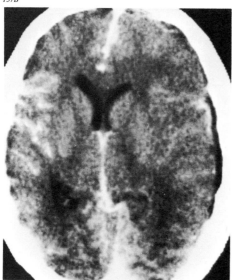

137B

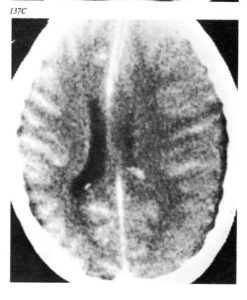

137C

The CT pattern of herpes simplex encephalitis, however, is not characteristic and can be seen in bacterial and other forms of encephalitis. Bacterial encephalitis may produce a mass effect, with a ventricular shift, gyral enhancement, and a low density zone in the temporal lobe, findings indistinguishable from those of herpes simplex encephalitis (fig. 137).

Besides viruses, the central nervous system may be affected by various other agents, including fungi (aspergillosis, candidiasis, cryptococcosis, coccidiodomycosis, histoplasmosis, blastomycosis, mucormycosis, nocardiosis, and actinomycosis); parasites (toxoplasmosis, cysticercosis, schistosomiasis, paragonimiasis and hydatidosis due to echninococci); and bacteria (tuberculosis, syphilis). The CT appearance of changes secondary to various infectious processes may be similar and nonspecific. For instance, multiple enhanced nodular or ring-like masses seen in toxoplasmosis and cysticercosis may simulate metastases or abscesses (fig. 138). Nodular enhancement seen in tuberculoma may resemble granuloma seen in sarcoidosis. Clinical history and laboratory findings are essential. Occasionally, histologic verification may be the only means for a final diagnosis (fig. 139).

Spectrum of CT Findings in Meningitis

The CT findings in meningitis vary a great deal. They include acute swelling, widening of the basal cisterns, interhemispheric fissure, and subarachnoid convexity space, ventricular widening, subdural collections, focal cortical necrosis, cerebral infarcts secondary to vasculitis, contrast enhancement of basal meninges, ventriculitis (ependymitis), as well as generalized cerebral atrophy (*Stovring and Snyder, 1980; Zimmerman et al. 1978*) (figs. 140–145).

Extracerebral collections are the most frequent abnormality demonstrated by CT and may be found as early as the third day of illness. A subdural tap probably is not necessary, unless there is a significant mass effect with ventricular shift.

Ependymitis may lead to irregularity of the contour of the ependymal lining of the lateral ventricle, which is detectable on CT. Enhancement of the meninges is a nonspecific sign and may be seen in granulomatous meningitis, as well as in acute bacterial meningitis. Ventricular dilatation

Fig. 137. Bacterial encephalitis in an 18-year-old male.

A Postcontrast scan showing large mass effect in the left frontotemporal region. The left frontal and temporal horns are completely obliterated, compared with the right ones.

B and C Marked ventricular shift to the right side with compression of the enhanced gyri as compared with the right hemisphere. The CT appearance of this case is indistinguishable from that of herpes simplex encephalitis (courtesy of Dr. LeRoy M. Kotzen).

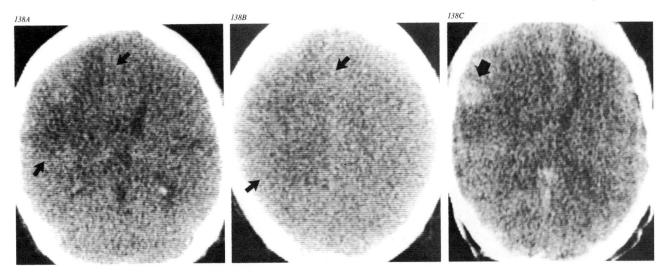

Fig. 138. Toxoplasmosis. This 40-year-old male with a 9-month history of weight loss and malaise was admitted 6 months ago with lymphadenopathy and negative biopsy of the nodes. Ten days before admission he developed intermittent slurred speech. Two days ago, on the day of admission, he had left arm drift followed by a grand mal seizure.

A and B Precontrast scans showing large low attenuation mass involving the right frontal, temporal, and parietal lobes (*arrows*) with marked compression of the right frontal horn and contralateral ventricular shift.

C and D Postcontrast scans showing three enhanced nodules, one in the right frontoparietal region near the cortex (*arrows*), one in the right posterior parietal lobe near the midline (*arrows*), and one in the right inferior frontal lobe (not shown).

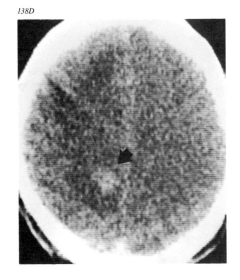

Fig. 139. Noncaseating granuloma with enhanced nodule in a 51-year-old black woman who, for 1 year, had episodic right frontal headache, scintilating scotomas in the left visual field, nausea, and rectal urgency. Several episodes were followed by loss of consciousness or impaired vision in the left visual field and at least one clonic seizure, which involved the left face, arm, and leg. Neurologic examinations were normal except for a left homonymous hemianopia that resolved after several hours. The cerebrospinal fluid was normal except for a protein of 60 mg percent. Precontrast scan (not shown here) revealed a low attenuation lesion in the right occipital and posterior parietal region.

A and B Postcontrast scans reveal a well-defined, homogenously enhanced nodular lesion in the occipital lobe surrounded by a considerable amount of edema. A right carotid arteriogram revealed an avascular mass in the parietooccipital area. Subtotal resection was performed and pathologically a nonceaseating granuloma was found. No acid-fast bacillus was found or cultured from the brain tissue. The appearance of the nodular lesion on CT cannot be differentiated from that of intracranial tuberculoma.

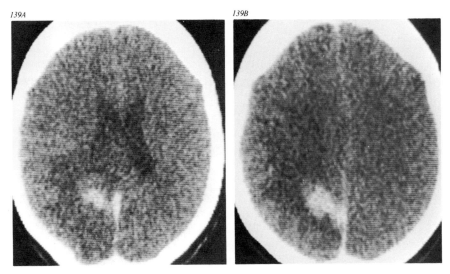

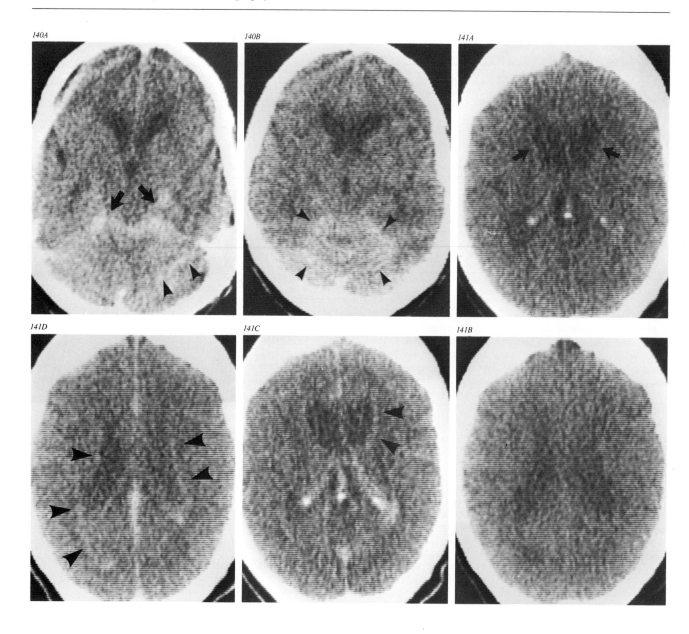

is another common abnormality secondary to meningitis seen on CT.

Rarely is diffuse necrosis of subcortical white matter seen following bacterial meningitis. There changes are attributed to various degrees of edema, vasculitis, foci of hemorrhage, and ischemic infarction.

Progressive Multifocal Leukoencephalopathy (PML)

This disease is a progressive demyelinating condition primarily affecting immunologically compromised patients and patients afflicted with chronic lymphocytic leukemia, or Hodgkin disease. Papova (papilloma-polyoma-vacuolating) viruses have been found in patients with PML. The condition involves primarily the white matter of the cerebral

Fig. 140.   A and B   An example of purulent bacterial meningitis with postcontrast enhancement of the perimesencephalic cisterns (*arrows*), the subarachnoid spaces around the tentorium, and the cerebellar and vermian cisterns (*arrowheads*). The CT appearance is indistinguishable from that of carcinomatous meningitis.

Fig. 141.   An example of ventriculitis.

A and B   Precontrast scans demonstrate a moderate degree of ventricular enlargement with a faint rim of increased attenuation around the walls of the frontal horns (*arrows*).

C and D   Postcontrast scans reveal marked enhancement of the ependyma outlining the walls of both lateral ventricles (*arrowheads*).

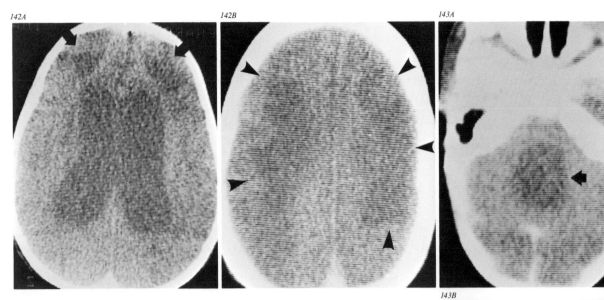

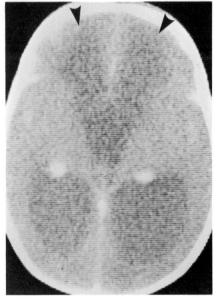

Fig. 142. Communicating hydrocephalus in a 1-year-old boy, a known case of spastic quadriplegia secondary to *Haemophilus influenzae* meningitis at the age of 8 months.

A Postcontrast scan showing a marked degree of communicating hydrocephalus with ventricular dilatation. Well-defined low attenuation lesions (*arrows*) were noted in the brain parenchyma of both frontal lobes anterior to the frontal horns, probably representing encephalomalacia and atrophy. The etiology of frontal lobe predilection is not known.

B Postcontrast scan showing extensive encephalomalacia involving the brain parenchyma above the lateral ventricles on both sides (*arrowheads*).

Fig. 143. Postmeningitis communicating hydrocephalus with ballooned fourth ventricle and periventricular lucency around the frontal horns. This 5-week-old female infant, status post *E. Coli* sepsis and meningitis, developed seizures 2½ weeks ago. The patient now presents with bulging fontanelles and rapidly increasing head circumference.

A Postcontrast scan reveals hugely dilated fourth ventricle (*arrows*) and occipital horns.

B Marked communicating hydrocephalus with periventricular lucencies anterior to the frontal horns (*arrowheads*). Periventricular lucency of various degrees has often been observed in the frontal horn when the hydrocephalus has progressed to an advanced stage. The low density zone is thought to represent acute periventricular edema, caused by the shift of water from the ventricle due to the increased intraventricular pressure.

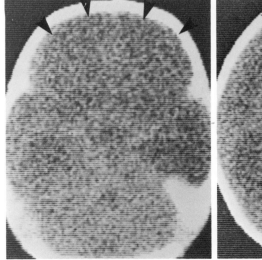

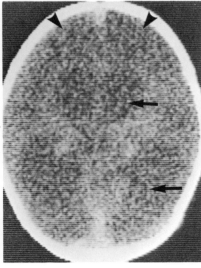

Fig. 144. A case of severe frontal lobe leukomalacia following meningitis in a 5½-week-old female infant who was admitted because of tremor and jerky movement. The patient had a history of acute bacterial meningitis at one week of age and was critically ill with apnea.

A Postcontrast scan shows normal fourth ventricle and surrounding posterior fossa structure. Large areas of abnormally decreased attenuation involves the brain parenchyma of both frontal lobes (*arrowheads*).

B Disproportionate dilatation of the frontal and occipital horns (*arrows*). Severe leukomalacia anterior to the frontal horns is detectable (*arrowhead*).

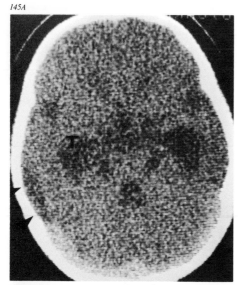

145A

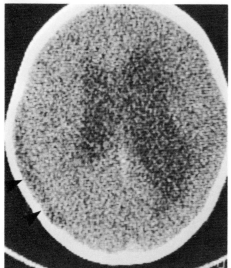

145B

Fig. 145. An example of subdural effusion and hydrocephalus in an 8-month-old infant as a complication 3 weeks postmeningitis.

A and B Postcontrast scans reveal chronic subdural effusion (*arrowheads*) causing compression of the dilated lateral ventricle. The right transverse sinus is normally enhanced (*arrows*). The temporal horns (T) and the fourth ventricle are markedly dilated.

Fig. 146. Progressive multifocal leukoencephalopathy in a 46-year-old white woman with a history of endstage renal disease. She was on hemodialysis, immunosuppressive therapy, and status-post lateral renal donor transplant. She was admitted for drooping of the left eyelid, intention tremor of the left arm, weakness of the legs, and broad-based gait. Physical examination revealed a left-sided upper motor neuron lesion. Lumbar puncture yielded clear CSF with 73 mg/dl protein and 74 mg/dl glucose. Relevant laboratory intestigations revealed relative polymorphonuclear leukopenia, lymphopenia, anemia, uremia, elevated creatinine, and elevated serum enzymes.

A to C Postcontrast scans reveal low attenuation lesion confined to the white matter of the left frontal lobe (*arrows*). The lesion does not conform to the territory of an arterial supply and stops abruptly at the subcortical gray-white junction. Another low density lesion is noted in the left cerebellar hemisphere (*arrowheads*). Both lesions are not enhanced by contrast medium and do not show changes on follow-up CT 11 days later. The patient underwent nephrectomy of the transplant, and postoperatively she developed left sided pneumothorax, increased respiratory secretions, hypotension, and GI bleeding associated with rapid deterioration of her neurologic status, culminating in death on the 15th postoperative day. Autopsy revealed lesions in the frontal, temporo-occipital regions of the left cerebral hemisphere, cerebellum, and brain stem, which were confined to the white matter. The histologic features of the lesions were consistent with progressive multifocal leukoencephalopathy. The electron microscopic examination revealed intranuclear virions, consistent with Papova virus of progressive multifocal leukoencephalopathy.

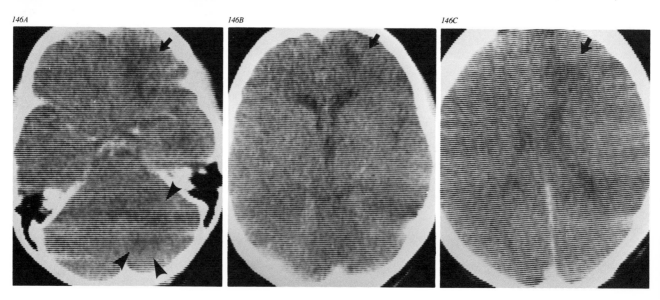

146A   146B   146C

hemispheres. Death usually occurs between 3 to 6 months following the onset of symptoms. Diagnostic tests in PML are usually negative. Cerebrospinal fluid examination is almost always normal, except for an occasional mild elevation of protein.

CT scans demonstrate characteristic low-density lesions confined in the white matter without a mass effect or contrast enhancement. White matter low density lesions may show characteristic scalloped periphery borders and may enlarge on subsequent scans. These scalloped lateral borders follow the contours of the subcortical gray-line junction. The areas of involvement do not follow the cerebral blood vessel distribution, as in infarction (fig. 146).

Bibliography

Benton JR, Wilson GH, Helmer E, et al: Computed tomography in intracranial cysticercosis. J Comput Assist Tomogr 1:464, 1977.

Brown, W, Zimmerman RA, Bilaniuk LT: Polycystic brain disease complicating neonatal meningitis: documentation of evolution by computed tomography. J Pediatr 94:757, 1979.

Carroll BA, Lane B, Norman D, et al: Diagnosis of progressive multifocal leukoencephalopathy by computed tomography. Radiology 122:137, 1977.

Cockrill Jr HH, Dreisbach J, Lowe B, et al: Computed tomography in leptomeningeal infections. AJR 130:511, 1978.

Danziger A. Price H, Schechter MM: An analysis of 113 intracranial infections. Neuroradiology 19:31, 1980.

Davis JM, Davis KR, Kleinman GM, et al: Computed tomography of herpes simplex encephalitis, with clinicopathological correlation. Radiology 129:409, 1978.

Dublin AB, Merten DF: Computed tomography in the evaluation of herpes simplex encephalitis. Radiology 125:133, 1977.

Dubois PJ, Martinez AJ, Myerowitz RA, et al: subependymal and leptomeningeal spread of systemic malignant lymphoma demonstrated by computed tomography. J Comput Assist Tomogr 2:217, 1978.

Enzmann DR, Brant-Zawadzki M, Britt RH: CT of central nervous system infections in immunocompromised patients. AJR 135:263, 1980.

Enzmann DR, Norman D, Mani J, et al: Computed tomography of granulomatous basal arachnoiditis. Radiology 120:341, 1976.

Enzmann DR, Ranson B, Norman D, et al: Computed tomography of herpes simplex encephalitis. Radiology 129:419, 1978.

Kalsbeck JE, DeSousa AL, Kleiman B, et al: Compartmentalization of the cerebral ventricles of a sequela of neonatal meningitis. J Neurosurg 52:547, 1980.

Karandanis D, Shulman JA: Factors associated with mortality in brain abscess. Arch Intern Med 135:1145, 1975.

Kaufman DM, Zimmerman RD, Leeds NE: Computed tomography in herpes simplex encephalitis. Neurology 29:1392, 1979.

Lott T, El Gammal T, Desilva R, et al: Evaluation of brain and epidural abscesses by computed tomography. Radiology 122:371, 1977.

Low JS, Weiner RL, Lin JP, et al: Computed tomography in herpes simplex encephalitis. Surg Neurol 10:313, 1978.

Luken III MG, Whelan MA: Recent diagnostic experience with subdural emphyema. J Neurosurg 52:764, 1980.

McGahan JP, Graves DS, Palmer PES, et al: Classic and contemporary imaging of coccidioidomycosis. AJR 136:793, 1961.

McGeachie RE, Gold LHA, Latchaw RE: Periventricular spread of tumor demonstrated by computed tomography. Radiology 125:407, 1977.

Mervis B, Lotz JW: Computed tomography in parenchymatous cerebral cysticercosis. Clin Radiol 31:521, 1981.

Nielsen H, Gyldensted C: Computed tomography in the diagnosis of cerebral abscess. Neuroradiology 12:207, 1977.

Peatfield RC, Shawdon HH: Five cases of intracranial tuberculoma followed by serial computerized tomography. J Neurol Neurosurg Psychiatry 42:373, 1979.

Sadhu VK, Handel SF, Pinto RS, et al: Neuroradiologic diagnosis of subdural empyema and CT limitations. AJNR 1:39, 1980.

Salmon JH: Ventriculitis complicating meningitis. Am J Dis Child 4:211, 1980.

Schultz P, Leeds NE: Intraventricular septations complicating neonatal meningitis. J Neurosurg 38:620, 1973.

Stovring J, Snyder RD: Computed tomography in childhood bacterial meningitis. J Pediatr 96:820, 1980.

Whelan MA, Hilal SK: Computed tomography as a guide in the diagnosis and follow-up of brain abscesses. Radiology 135:663, 1980.

Whelan MA, Stern J: Intracranial tuberculoma. Radiology 138:75, 1981.

Zee CS, Segall HD, Miller C, et al: Unusual neuroradiological features of intracranial cysticercosis. Radiology 137:397, 1980.

Zimmerman RA, Patel S, Bilaniuk L: Demonstration of purulent bacterial intracranial infections by computed tomography. AJR 127:155, 1976.

Zimmerman RD, Russell EJ, Leeds NE, et al: Computed tomography in the early diagnosis of herpes simplex encephalitis. AJR 134:61, 1980.

Suggested Reading

Alfidi RJ, Haaga J, Weinstein M, et al: Computed Tomography of the Human Body: An Atlas of Normal Anatomy. CV Mosby, St Louis, 1977

Binder GA, Haughton VM, Ho KC: Computed Tomography of the Brain in Axial, Coronal and Sagittal Planes. Little, Brown, Boston, 1979

Carter B, Morehead J, Wolpert SM, et al: Cross-Sectional Anatomy: Computed Tomography and Ultrasound Correlation. Appleton-Century-Crofts, New York, 1977

Eycleshymer AC, Schoemaker DM: A Cross-Section Anatomy. Appleton-Century-Crofts, New York, 1939

Gonzalez CF, Grossman CF, Palacios E: Computed Brain and Orbital Tomography: Technique and Interpretation. Wiley, New York, 1976

Hanaway J, Scott WR, Strother CM: Atlas of the Human Brain and the Orbit for Computed Tomography. Green, St Louis, 1977

Henderson SD: Pathology in Computed Tomography of the Brain. CC Thomas, Springfield, Illinois, 1978

Jabbour J, Ramey DR, Roach S: Atlas of C. T. Scans in Pediatric Neurology. Medical Examination Publishing Company, Flushing, New York, 1977

Jacobs L, Jones JM, D'agostino A: Computerized Tomography of the Orbit and Sella Turcica. Raven Press, New York, 1980

Laffey PL, Oaks WW, Swanmi RK, et al: Computerized Tomography in Clinical Medicine. Medical Direction, Philadelphia, 1976

Ledley RS, Huang HK, Mazziotta JC: Cross-Sectional Anatomy—an Atlas for Computerized Tomography. Williams and Wilkins, Baltimore, 1977

Matsui T, Hirano A: An Atlas of the Human Brain for Computerized Tomography. Igaku-Shoin, Tokyo, 1978

New PFJ, Scott WR: Computed Tomography of the Brain and Orbit (EMI Scanning). Williams and Wilkins, Baltimore, 1975

Norman D, Korobkin M, Newton TH: Computed Tomography, Mosby, St Louis, 1977

Oldendorf WH: The Quest for an Image of Brain: Computerized Tomography in the Perspective of Past and Future Imaging Methods. Raven Press, New York, 1980

Pernkopf E: Atlas of Topographical and Applied Human Anatomy, Vol 1. WB Saunders, Philadelphia, 1963

Potter GD: Sectional Anatomy and Tomography of the Head. Grune and stratton, New York, 1971

Ramsey RG: Computed Tomography of the Brain with Clinical, Angiographic, and Radionuclide Correlation. WB Saunders, Philadelphia, 1977

Roberts M, Hanaway J: Atlas of the Human Brain in Section. Lea and Febiger, Philadelphia, 1970

Shipps FC: Atlas of Brain Anatomy for C. T. Scans, Using EMI Terminology. CC Thomas, Springfield, Illinois, 1977

Taveras J, Wood E: Diagnostic Neuroradiology. Williams and Wilkins, Baltimore, 1976

Weisberg LA, Nice C, Katz M: Cerebral Computed Tomography: a Text-Atlas. WB Saunders, Philadelphia, 1978

Index

Figure numbers are set in *italics*. Page numbers are in roman type.